SEE Your Way to Better Health

Donald J. Mertens

VANTAGE Press
New York

"Stop Questionnaire: A Tool to Screen patients...," reprinted by permission of Wolters Kluwer, a division of Lippincott Williams & Wilkins. All rights reserved.

Epworth Sleepiness Scale, reprinted by permission of the Sleep Research Society, © American Academy of Sleep Medicine. All rights reserved.

Each individual should seek the advice of his or her own physician before starting any new medical program. The opinions and instructions expressed herein are solely those of the author.

FIRST EDITION

Published by Vantage Press, Inc.
419 Park Ave. South, New York, NY 10016

Manufactured in the United States of America
ISBN: 978-0-533-16340-3

Library of Congress Catalog Card No: 2010900543

0 9 8 7 6 5 4 3 2 1

Contents

Acknowledgments

I would like to thank Fran Berkoff for reviewing the chapter on eating and for her helpful criticism and suggestions, and Dr. Harley Smythe for reviewing the endocrine and sleep chapters.

I also thank my children for their help with the diagrams and pictures, and for their support for the project.

Introduction

SEE represents the three pillars on which good health rests; adequate Sleep, regular Exercise and Eating the right food in appropriate quantity. A great deal has been written about all three, but no one seems to have put them all together.

Canada's food guide addresses eating, and Participaction addresses exercise, but sleep is rarely mentioned as an important factor for good health, and yet all three are intimately connected. Approximately half of all diseases in developed countries are lifestyle related. An old Chinese saying states that a superior doctor prevents disease, a good doctor treats disease before it is evident and a mediocre doctor treats the full-blown disease. Hippocrates (46–370 B.C.) said that if we could give every individual the right amount of nourishment and exercise, not too little and not too much, we would have found the safest way to health. So we see that the idea of a healthy lifestyle and disease prevention is not new, just neglected.

The pressures of living in a modern industrial society require long hours of work to earn a living and look after a family. Time is constrained such that for most people it is difficult to live a healthy lifestyle even with the best of intentions. Additionally physical activity is being engineered out of our daily lives, so we need to set aside time specifically to be physically active, which most of us do not do.

As we look for more time to accomplish our daily tasks, the first thing to suffer is usually sleep. Going to bed an hour or two later, or rising an hour earlier is the simplest way to find more time, but unfortunately leads to sleep deprivation, which in turn adversely affects our health and productivity. Sleep deprivation is linked to the development of the metabolic syndrome, diabetes and the epidemic of obesity that is currently afflicting the world's populations.

Another way that we find extra time, is to eat pre-prepared and/or fast foods, which often are loaded with saturated fats and excessive amounts of salt, leading to obesity, diabetes, coronary artery disease and high blood pressure.

I have spent many years working in cardiac rehabilitation. This is a very rewarding field, and it is very gratifying to see people who have had a heart attack or heart surgery regain their confidence, and become active again, often ending up being much fitter than they were before their illness, but how much better to have prevented their problem in the first place. Your inherited genes, which make you susceptible to various illnesses, cannot be changed, but they only load the gun, it is your lifestyle that pulls the trigger.

In this book I attempt to set out some of what is known about sleep, exercise and nutrition, with regard to health and performance, in the hope that this understanding may encourage some of you to adopt a healthy lifestyle and improve your quality of life. I know from personal experience how much better and younger one feels, and how much more productive one is when following SEE.

SEE Your Way to Better Health

1

The Endocrine System

Sleep, eating and exercise all impact on the endocrine system and vice versa, so an understanding of the basic components and functions of the system are necessary to an understanding of the role played by the three pillars of healthy living.

The endocrine system is comprised of a number of different glands that produce chemical messengers called hormones that are transported by the circulatory system to target cells in other parts of the body. Target cells have receptors that are specific to the messenger hormones that bind the hormones to the cell, and produce a response. Cells that do not have the specific receptors therefore do not respond.

The endocrine system acts with the nervous system to coordinate the body's activities. The hypothalamus is a part of the brain and is the pathway that links the brain with the endocrine system. It is responsible for maintaining constant internal conditions by regulating the internal environment. It achieves this by regulating heart rate, body temperature, water balance, and the secretions of the pituitary gland.

The following glands make up the endocrine system.

Pituitary and pineal in the brain
Thyroid and parathyroid in the neck

Thymus in the chest
Adrenal and pancreas, in the abdomen
Ovaries in the female and testes in the male

Several other body organs also produce hormones, including the heart, lungs, liver, stomach, intestines, kidneys, fat cells and skin.

The pineal gland produces melatonin that promotes sleep, responding to light stimulating the optic nerves. It produces melatonin in response to darkness and shuts down in response to bright light.

The pituitary gland consists of an anterior and posterior lobe. The posterior lobe releases oxytocin and antidiuretic hormone (ADH), hormones that are synthesized in the neurons of the hypothalamus and stored in the pituitary gland. Oxytocin stimulates uterine contractions during childbirth and secretion of milk from the breast after childbirth. ADH promotes reabsorption of water in the tubules of the kidney, thereby helping to regulate the amount of fluid in the body and the amount of urine produced.

The anterior lobe of the pituitary produces six different hormones, three that stimulate the thyroid, adrenal cortex and the sex glands (ovaries and testes), and three that have direct effects on the body, growth hormone, prolactin and melanocyte stimulating hormones. Growth hormone stimulates the cells of the body to grow. If too little is produced dwarfism results, and if too much is produced gigantism is the result. Growth hormone is also involved in the repair of body tissues, and is largely released during sleep. Prolactin is produced in large quantities after childbirth and stimulates the development of glandular breast tissue and milk production. It is also involved in the metabolism of fats and carbohydrates.

Melanocyte stimulating hormone causes the melano-

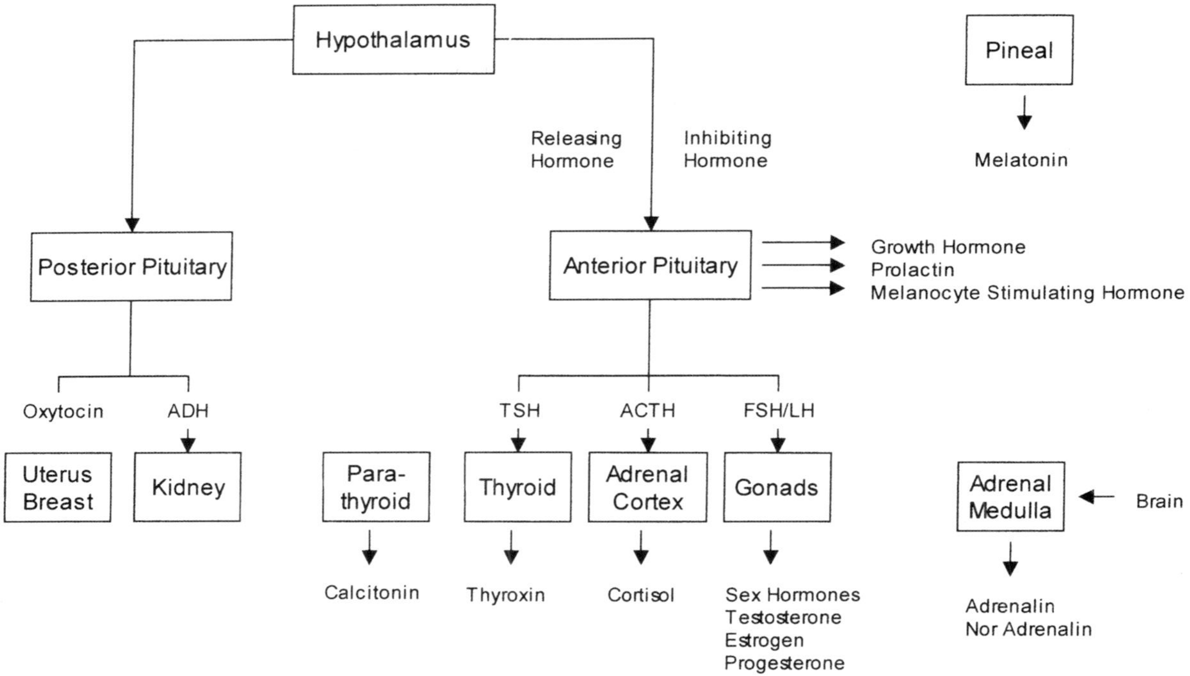

Figure 1. Diagram of components of the endocrine system.

cytes to produce melanin, a pigment in the skin that helps to protect us from the harmful rays of the sun. melanin gives moles their brown color and is responsible for the darkening of the skin called suntan. Thyroid Stimulating Hormone causes the thyroid gland to produce thyroxin (T4) and triiodothyronine (T3). Both have similar effects on target cells influencing metabolic rate, growth and development.

Too little thyroxin in adults results in lethargy and weight gain, but in infants causes dwarfism, mental retardation and lack of sexual maturity (cretinism). Too much thyroxin increases heart rate and blood pressure and results in weight loss and tremor.

Thyroxin production is regulated by a negative feedback mechanism; thyroxin inhibits the hypothalamus and the pituitary gland from further stimulating the thyroid gland. Hormone secretions by glands controlled by the hypothalamus are regulated by a negative feedback mechanism. When the hormone levels are high, they inhibit the hypothalamus and anterior pituitary, resulting in a decline in their levels.

Iodine is required for the manufacture of thyroid hormones. A deficiency causes lack of thyroxin production and subsequently failure of the negative feedback mechanism, resulting in excess production of thyroid stimulating hormone by the pituitary gland, that in turn causes enlargement of the thyroid gland, commonly known as a goiter. Goiters used to be much more common, but the addition of iodine to table salt has largely eliminated the problem.

The thyroid gland also produces calcitonin, a hormone that stimulates calcium deposition in bones Production of calitonin is regulated by the level of calcium in the blood and not by the pituitary gland. When the level of calcium is high, calcitonin production is stimulated.

Parathyroid Hormone (PTH) is produced in the para-

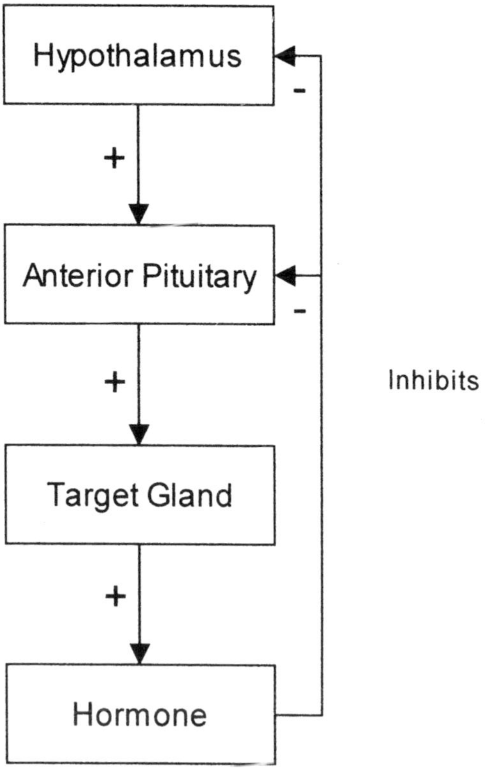

Figure 2. Diagram of negative feedback

thyroid glands, four small glands found on the back of the thyroid gland. PTH acts to increase the level of calcium in the blood by stimulating calcium removal from bones and by causing the kidneys to increase the reabsorption of calcium. It also activates vitamin D which increases the absorption of calcium from ingested food.

Adrenocorticotropin (ACTH) stimulates the adrenal cortex to produce Cortisol. Cortisol is known as a glucocorticoid hormone because it raises the level of glucose in the blood by stimulating the liver to produce and release glucose. Typically this occurs in response to stress. The adrenal cortex also produces Aldosterone, known as a mineralocorticoid hormone. It acts on the kidney to stimulate the kidney to conserve sodium and excrete potassium. Increased sodium in the blood retains water and increases the volume of blood in the vascular system. The production of Aldosterone is not controlled by the pituitary gland. If the body senses that there is too much blood, the heart produces Atrial Naturetic Peptide, which suppresses the release of Aldosterone from the adrenal cortex, causing the kidney to excrete more sodium. It also inhibits the release of Antidiuretic Hormone thereby stimulating the kidney to excrete more water.

The adrenal medulla is composed of modified nerve cells that secrete Epinephrine and Norepinephrine (Adrenaline and Noradrenalin). Their secretion is controlled by centers in the brain, including the hypothalamus, via sympathetic nerves. Because their release is stimulated through the nervous system rather than the circulatory system, the response is much quicker. These hormones are released in response to stress, increasing the heart rate, the level of glucose in the blood, and directing the blood flow from the skin to the muscles (pallor and cold sweat) in preparation for action. These changes are sometimes referred to as the fright, fight or flight response, and developed in order to improve our chances of survival in dangerous situations. If you have ever experienced a severe fright you will no doubt recognize the symptoms just described.

Luteinizing Hormone ((LH) released from the anterior pituitary gland has different effects on males and females. In males it stimulates the testes to produce male hormones known as androgens, one of which is testosterone. In females it stimulates the ovaries to produce the female hormones estrogen and progesterone.

These hormones are responsible for the development of secondary sex characteristics at puberty. In males deepening the voice, development of pubic, axillary and facial hair and increase in muscle mass. In females breast development, widening of the pelvis and growth of pubic and axillary hair. Both sexes develop increased activity of sweat and sebaceous glands that may in some, result in acne.

Follicle Stimulating Hormone (FSH) also from the anterior pituitary controls egg and sperm production.

The pancreas, situated within the abdominal cavity, is connected by the pancreatic duct to the duodenum, and produces enzymes that help us to digest our food. Within the pancreas there are groups of specialized cells called the islets of Langerhans. These cells produce two hormones called insulin and glucagon.

Insulin promotes the removal of glucose from the blood and helps to get it into the muscles and liver. It also is necessary for the process of converting excess glucose into fat for storage, and is involved in the production of muscle protein. If there is insufficient insulin, or insulin resistance, the body is unable to use glucose, and diabetes develops. Glucagon is also produced in the islets of Langerhans, but by different cells. The effect of glucagon is the opposite of insulin. It raises the level of glucose in the blood by releasing it from body stores, and is usually released between meals to maintain an adequate level of glucose in the blood.

The thymus gland lies within the chest cavity and plays a part in the immune system's functioning. White blood cells called lymphocytes are cells that help to fight infection. There are two kinds, B cells and T cells. The hormone produced by the thymus stimulates the development of T cells that participate in recognizing and destroying infected cells within the body.

The stomach produces a hormone called ghrelin, which stimulates appetite. The intestine produces two hormones that are known as incretins. Incretins stimulate insulin release from the pancreas and slow the rate of absorption of nutrients by reducing the rate of gastric emptying. They also inhibit the release of glucagon.

The kidney secretes two hormones, erythropoietin (EPO) and calcitriol. EPO stimulates the bone marrow to produce more red blood cells that carry oxygen around the body. When moving from sea level to altitude, where there is less oxygen in the air, the kidney produces more EPO and there is an increase in the number of red blood cells to help the body cope with the decreased oxygen. Athletes have used EPO to try to gain a competitive advantage by increasing the number of red blood cells, in an effort to get more oxygen to their muscles during competition. Doping with EPO is considered cheating, and if discovered leads to disqualification. Athletes have also trained at altitude in an attempt to get the same effect, but the results have been disappointing in terms of enhanced performance. EPO is often used as a medication for people who have kidney failure.

Calcitriol is manufactured from calciferol (vitamin D3), which is synthesized in the skin when it is exposed to sunlight. Calcitriol helps the intestine to absorb calcium and releases calcium from bones into the blood.

The heart makes two hormones, A-type and B-type natriuretic peptide, both of which help to lower blood pressure by relaxing small blood vessels, inhibiting aldosterone, and helping the kidney to get rid of more sodium.

Fat cells also produce hormones, Leptin being an example. Leptin has the effect of decreasing appetite.

This has been a brief and simplified summary of the

endocrine system that will hopefully make the following chapters easier to understand.

> The endocrine system connects the brain and the body.
> The pituitary gland is the conductor of the endocrine orchestra.
> The system functions to coordinate bodily activities.

2
Sleep

Sleep may be defined as a natural periodic state of rest for the mind and body, in which the eyes usually close and consciousness is completely or partially lost, accompanied by a decrease in bodily movement and responsiveness to external stimuli.

Sleep onset and offset are determined by a biological clock called a circadian rhythm. The term circadian is derived from the Latin Circa, about, and Diem, day, meaning approximately one day, corresponding to the rotation of the earth (24 hours). The circadian rhythm is generated within the brain, by specialized cells in the suprachiasmatic nuclei (SCN) located in the hypothalamus. The SCN receives information about illumination from the eyes. The SCN communicates that information to the pineal gland that in turn secretes the hormone melatonin. The circadian rhythm can be altered by external factors called Zeitgerbers, the most important being daylight.

Sleep is divided into two types. Rapid eye movement (REM) and non-rapid eye movement sleep (NREM), each type is associated with different physiological, neurological and psychological features. NREM sleep is divided into four phases, each phase characterized by distinctive brain wave patterns as measured by electroencephalograpy (EEG). The EEG records the electrical impulses (waves) in the brain, in the same way that an electrocardiogram (ECG) records the electrical activity in the heart muscle. Heart rate, breathing rate, blood pressure and muscle tone are all reduced during NREM sleep.

During stage one, which is light sleep, we drift in and out of sleep and can be easily aroused. When we enter stage two our eye movements stop and our brain waves become slower, with occasional bursts of rapid waves called sleep spindles. In stage three extremely slow brain waves (delta waves) appear, interspersed with smaller faster waves. In stage four the brain waves are almost exclusively delta waves. Stages three and four are associated with deep sleep and it is difficult to awaken the subject, who may feel groggy and disoriented for a few minutes after being roused.

During stage five (REM sleep), breathing becomes more rapid, shallow and irregular, and there are associated rapid, jerky eye movements with temporary paralysis of the limb muscles. Heart rate and blood pressure increases, and males may develop penile erections.

Sleep occurs in cycles of NREM and REM, with the order usually being NREM stage one, stage two, stage three, stage four and then REM. Each complete cycle lasts between 90 to 100 minutes. The first sleep cycles each night contain relatively short REM periods and long periods of deep sleep. As the night progresses, REM sleep periods increase in length, while deep sleep decreases. REM sleep accounts for about 20 to 25% of total sleep and is the time when dreaming occurs.

Timing of sleep is determined by circadian rhythm, biochemistry and by willed behavior. A chemical called adenosine builds up in the blood through the day, and high levels cause drowsiness. As a result of the circadian rhythm the brain releases melatonin, and the body temperature decreases, producing a feeling of sleepiness.

The amount of sleep required varies with age, being higher in the very young and gradually decreasing as we age. Babies will average 18 hours per day; adolescents seem to need 9–10 per day, and adults 7–9 hours per day. A 2003 study from the University of Pennsylvania School of Medicine found that cognitive performance in adults declined with less than 8 hours of sleep per night.

Sleep is a basic requirement for life and sleep deprivation if severe enough can cause death. Sleep is needed to restore and keep brain metabolic functioning healthy. Sleep deprivation can be due to medical disorders such as sleep apnea, alcohol and substance abuse, depression or due to an unbalanced lifestyle.

Sleep Apnea

Sleep apnea is a sleep disorder characterized by pauses in breathing during sleep. A minimum of five episodes per hour, lasting at least ten seconds is required to establish the diagnosis. Episodes are associated with brief neurological arousal and or, a fall in the level of oxygen in the blood. There are tree types of sleep apnea, obstructive, central and mixed.

Central sleep apnea is due to a failure of the central controlling area of the brain called the respiratory center, which is situated in the lower part of the brain stem. In severe cases, a person suffering from this problem is reliant on a machine for breathing and will die without mechanical assistance. This condition is called Ondine's Curse. Ondine was a mythical water nymph that fell in love with a mortal, a dashing knight called Sir Lawrence. Water nymphs are immortal, but if they bear a mortal's child they lose their immortality and gain a soul. Ondine and Sir Lawrence married and on his wedding day Lawrence vowed "My every waking breath shall be a pledge of love and faithfulness to you." One year later Ondine gave birth to Lawrence's child, and from that moment began to age. As Ondine's physical attractiveness diminished, Lawrence lost interest in his wife. One day Ondine found him asleep, snoring, in the arms of another woman. Ondine woke him up and uttered a curse: "You swore faithfulness to me with every waking breath and I accepted your oath. So be it. As long as you are awake you shall have your breath, but should you fall asleep, then that breath shall be taken from you and you will die."

Obstructive sleep apnea is by far the most common form of sleep apnea, accounting for 84% of cases. The condition is estimated to affect one in every fifteen people, and is caused by collapse of the airway during sleep, especially when lying on one's back. Sometimes turning onto one side will relieve the problem. The diagnosis is made either in a sleep laboratory, or at home, using an oxygen sensor to measure the oxygen content of the blood during sleep.

If your sleeping partner complains that you snore and seem to stop breathing from time to time, and you wake up feeling tired and unrefreshed, you should suspect that you might suffer from obstructive sleep apnea, and discuss this with your doctor. Obstructive sleep apnea is more common in people with thick necks. A neck measuring more than 43cm, or collar size larger than 16.5 should raise suspicion, if any of the other symptoms listed above are present.

Obstructive sleep apnea is also a cause of having to get up more than once in the night to urinate (nocturia). Trying to breathe against a closed airway causes increased negative pressure in the chest cavity, which in turn causes increased filling of the heart, tricking it into believing that there is excessive fluid in the body. The heart then releases a hormone called atrial naturetic peptide that increases the production of urine in an effort to get rid of the excess fluid.

Sleep apnea is associated with an increased risk of heart disease, stroke, high blood pressure, insulin resistance and an increase in C reactive protein, a marker of inflammation. It is therefore not surprising that sleep disorders are very common in chronic inflammatory diseases such as arthritis.

Sleep apnea is also associated with, and may be a cause of gout. The reduction of oxygen secondary to apnea causes an increase in uric acid in the blood, and an associated increase in carbon dioxide, increasing the acidity of the blood, which promotes the formation of uric acid crystals, causing gout, a form of arthritis.

Recent research published in the June 2008 edition of *Neuroscience* letters, using magnetic resonance imaging, reported that people with obstructive sleep apnea show tissue loss in brain regions that are associated with memory.

Many drugs act on the brain to depress the respiratory center, including alcohol, opiates, barbiturates, benzodiazepines, and many other tranquilizers, all can cause or exacerbate sleep apnea.

I well remember a line worker at General Motors, who was attending the health center with increasing frequency due to feeling light headed and dizzy. She would present looking pale and sweaty, with low blood pressure. She felt constantly tired and without energy, had difficulty concentrating and eventually was having trouble managing her family chores, as well as her work. She was referred for investigations, but all her test results came back normal, until it was discovered that she had severe sleep apnea. After a period of treatment with constant positive airway pressure, all her symptoms disappeared and her energy returned. The unusual finding in this case was low blood pressure, as sleep apnea is usually associated with high blood pressure.

People with this condition awaken in the morning feeling tired, but unaware that their sleep has been disturbed, and may find themselves nodding off during the day. Treatment requires being connected to a machine, which uses positive pressure to keep the airway open (CPAP) while sleeping. Unfortunately many people find the equipment uncomfortable to use, and therefore compliance with this form of treatment can be a problem.

In 2005 a paper in the *British Medical Journal* reported that Didgeridoo playing improved symptoms of moderate obstructive sleep apnea. Subsequently a randomized controlled trial carried out in Brazil, and published in May 2008, has confirmed that oropharyngeal exercises can indeed improve symptoms in people suffering from obstructive sleep apnea.

Depression

Depression is associated with disordered sleeping. The majority of depressed people take longer to get to sleep, and have early awakening with difficulty getting back to sleep. Some depressed people, about 15%, oversleep and have trouble getting out of bed. In the past it was thought that depression was the cause of the sleep disorder, but recently it has become apparent that lack of sleep may in fact be a precursor of depression. A study done at the University of Rochester's Sleep and Neurophysiology Research Laboratory found that seniors who were not depressed, but suffered from insomnia were six times more likely to be depressed at some point in their lives than seniors who did not have insomnia. Dr. Michael Perlis, the director of the lab, concluded that "What we know is that insomnia is a risk factor for depression, it precedes depression and it seems to make depression resistant to treatment."

A report on the Wisconsin Sleep Cohort Study published in the *Archives of Internal Medicine* in 2006 observed a significant dose response trends of increasing risk of depression with increasing sleep-related breathing disorder severity. This study was comprised of 1408 participants between the ages of 30 and 60 years of age, who underwent overnight sleep studies every four years.

Another study published in the *Journal of Obstetric Gynecologic and Neonatal Nursing* in 2008 compared the sleeping patterns of 46 postpartum women, half with symptoms of postpartum depression and half without. Sleep patterns were monitored for seven consecutive days. Results showed that mothers suffering from postpartum depression took longer to fall asleep and slept for shorter periods. The worse the sleep quality, the worse was their depression.

Sleep cycles are abnormal in depressed people, with less deep NREM sleep and earlier REM sleep, as well as more frequent awakenings during the night. As a result depressed people often do not feel refreshed or well rested on awakening. When treating depression it is therefore important to address the sleep disturbance.

I have no doubt from my own personal experience that sleep deprivation can cause depression. When I was an intern, we used to work very long hours with little sleep, and on one occasion after a long period of inadequate sleep, I was taking a history from a patient, when I suddenly experienced an overwhelming feeling of sadness which was so intense that I was unable to continue, and had to leave the room. After some time alone during which I cried, I was able to return and complete the history.

Coronary Artery Disease

It has been well documented that sleep apnea is associated with a higher incidence of coronary artery disease, but a recent study has found that simple sleep deprivation is also associated with an increased incidence of coronary calcification, which is an indicator of coronary artery disease. This study by King et al. published in the December 2008 issue of the *Journal of the American Medical Association* looked at 495 health people, ages 35 to 47, who did not have artery disease and who were followed for five years. At the beginning of the study, they all had a CT scan, and after five years the scan was repeated. The group as a whole averaged six hours of sleep a night. Only 6% of those getting seven hours of sleep or more per night had coronary calcification, 11% of those sleeping five to seven hours and 27% of those sleeping less than five hours had coronary calcification. The authors took into consideration other known risk factors for heart disease, including sleep apnea, cholesterol, blood pressure, body weight, diabetes and depression. Getting an extra hour of sleep appears to lower the risk of getting coronary artery disease by the same amount as lowering systolic blood pressure by 16 mm Hg.

A review article from the Mayo Clinic published in the October 2003 issue of the *Journal of the American Medical Association,* looked at 154 original investigations and reviews of sleep related breathing disorders. They concluded that obstructive sleep apnea is common, readily diagnosed and usually treatable. It frequently coexists undiagnosed in patients with cardiovascular disease, activates disease mechanisms known to elicit cardiac and vascular damage, and may be implicated in progression of cardiovascular disease and resistance to conventional therapeutic strategies.

Obstructive sleep apnea is associated with increased

sympathetic activation, vascular endothelial dysfunction, increased oxidative stress, inflammation, increased platelet stickiness and metabolic dysregulation, all of which are associated with increased risk of heart disease. Metabolic dysregulation may be the result of increased cortisol secretion by the adrenal glands resulting from sleep deprivation.

Sleep disordered breathing is also known to be associated with ventricular arrhythmias, which can lead to sudden death.

Stroke

There is no doubt that obstructive sleep apnea is associated with stroke. Some work suggests that it increased the risk of stroke independent of the known vascular and metabolic factors. A study by Urbano et al. published in the December 2008 *Journal of Applied Physiology* showed that subjects with obstructive sleep apnea had lower oxygen saturation and lower cerebral artery flow velocity than healthy controls and elevated blood pressure within the brain. Repeated fluctuations may eventually harm the brain's ability to modulate these changes and prevent damage to itself. Normally the brain is able to regulate its blood flow to meet its metabolic needs, even in the face of blood pressure changes. This ability is called cerebral autoregulation.

Most people who have suffered a stroke have sleep disorders, but whether this is the cause or the result of the stroke is unknown.

Treating obstructive sleep apnea with CPAP reduces blood pressure, but we do not know whether it reduces the incidence of stroke.

Fibromyalgia

Fibromyalgia continues to be a subject of debate among doctors, as to whether it is a physical or psychosocial condition. At the time of diagnosis 30 to 50% of fibromyalgia patients exhibit mood disorders, primarily depression, which in turn means that the majority of such patients do not have mood disorders. Recent research has demonstrated differences in inflammatory markers, specifically interleukin-8, and loss of grey matter in the brains of patients diagnosed with fibromyalgia. Patients with fibromyalgia all suffer from sleep disturbance, and the absence of sleep disturbance rules out the diagnosis. These patients also have a decreased pain threshold. The relationship between pain and sleep may well be reciprocal. Some studies suggest that impaired sleep may precede the pain symptoms, and in one study where investigators disturbed normal subjects with sound, during NREM (slow wave) sleep, the subjects developed symptoms similar to those of fibromyalgia. In a more recent study, three nights of interrupted NREM sleep led to a reduction in pain threshold along with fibromyalgia-like symptoms. It is therefore possible that the abnormalities of the central nervous system seen in fibromyalgia may arise from impaired sleep rather than the other way around. Patients with fibromyalgia spend more time awake, more time in bed without sleeping, and more time in stage one NREM sleep than do healthy subjects. The decreased stage three NREM sleep may explain why their sleep is not restorative and may account for imbalances in serotonin and insulin like growth factor as well as abnormalities in the hypothalamic-pituitary-adrenal axis. This also fits with the beneficial effects of the serotonin-norepinephrine reuptake inhibitors used in the pharmacological treatment of this condition.

Exercise is also helpful, probably because of its effect on

the hypothalamic-pituitary-adrenal axis, but more of that in the section on exercise.

Drugs

Drugs my be either depressants or stimulants. A discussion of them all is beyond the scope of this book, but the major and most commonly encountered ones are as follows.

Depressants

Alcohol is a depressant that has a direct effect on the brain, and makes sleep apnea worse. Patients with severe obstructive sleep apnea who consume two or more alcoholic drinks a day have a fivefold increased risk of having a fatigue-related traffic accident. Alcohol initially allows a person to fall asleep more quickly, but also disrupts sleep patterns. Alcohol consumed within an hour of bedtime disrupts the second half of the sleep period. The subject may sleep fitfully during the second half of sleep, awakening from dreams and then having difficulty getting back to sleep. This sleep disturbance may be followed by daytime fatigue and sleepiness. These changes tend to be more pronounced in the elderly, as the brain alcohol level is higher than in a younger person for the same dose. Bedtime alcohol intake in the elderly has been found to lead to unsteadiness in walking when getting up in the night, associated with an increase in falls and injuries.

Sleep disturbances are common in alcoholics and are often exacerbated during withdrawal. Withdrawal may be associated with severe sleep fragmentation and pronounced insomnia. Sleep may consist almost entirely of brief periods of REM, which may in turn be related to the hallucinations that some people experience during withdrawal.

Interestingly, infants of mothers who consumed at least one alcoholic drink per day during the first trimester of pregnancy, exhibit sleep disruptions and increased arousal, compared to infants who were not exposed to alcohol. Infants exposed to alcohol in breast milk fall asleep sooner; but sleep less than infants that are not exposed.

Barbiturates acts as a depressant on the brain, and in the past were used to aid patients with insomnia. Due to their high propensity for addiction and narrow range between therapeutic and toxic dosage, they have fallen into disfavor in the treatment of insomnia. Barbiturates are now primarily used in anesthesia and for the control of epileptic seizures. Benzodiazepines are now the drugs of choice for the treatment of anxiety and insomnia. Another commonly used over-the-counter drug that people use to help them sleep is an antihistamine called diphenhydramine. While the short-term use of a drug to aid in treating insomnia may be justified, it is important to determine what the cause of the sleep problem is, and to use nonpharmacological methods whenever possible.

Beta-blockers are commonly prescribed drugs for the treatment of high blood pressure and for people who have had heart attacks. Unfortunately they decrease the production of melatonin by the brain, and are associated with sleep disturbances such as vivid dreams, nightmares, increased waking and insomnia. If you experience these side effects, consult with your doctor. Sometimes a change of medication can relieve these symptoms.

Melatonin is a hormone produced in the brain by converting tryptophan to serotonin and then melatonin, which is released at night by the pineal gland to induce and maintain sleep. Melatonin may be taken orally as an aid to sleep, and is used to help combat sleep disturbance due to jet lag. This practice is controversial and the Civil Aviation Authority in Britain has banned its use by aircrew.

The release of melatonin is dependent on darkness, and exposure to bright light during the night interferes with this process. There is some epidemiological evidence to suggest that people who work night shifts have a higher incidence of breast and colon cancer, and it is thought that interference with melatonin release may be implicated.

Opioids such as morphine, heroin, oxycodone and methadone are all associated with sleep disorders. They can all produce central sleep apnea by depressing the respiratory center in the brain, and reduce the time spent in deep sleep and REM sleep.

Stimulants

Amphetamines, commonly known as speed, are used therapeutically to treat narcolepsy and attention deficit hyperactivity disorder. Unfortunately they are also used recreationally and for weight reduction. Amphetamine, Dextroamphetamine, and methamphetamine are the most commonly encountered examples of this drug class. Their side effects include decreased appetite (hence their use for weight reduction), anxiety, insomnia, stimulation and increased alertness. They are highly addictive and may cause permanent damage to the brain.

MDMA a designer drug commonly called ecstasy, is a particularly dangerous form of amphetamine. It is a party drug that is often used at raves and nightclubs, and has been associated with deaths. MDMA can cause the body temperature to become severely elevated, a condition known as hyperthermia, cause seizures, cardiac rhythm disturbances, liver damage, chemical imbalance in the blood (low sodium), and psychiatric disorders. It increases the serotonin levels in the brain and is associated with sleep disturbances, increasing wakefulness and decreasing REM sleep.

Caffeine is probably the most commonly used stimulant in the world. My observation is that most North Americans cannot start their day without their cup of coffee. Caffeine acts by slowing the action of the hormones in the brain that cause sleepiness, thereby increasing alertness. Melatonin production is suppressed and adrenaline production enhanced. Caffeine also increases dopamine levels in the same way that amphetamines do, which is what makes it addictive. People vary greatly in their sensitivity to the effects of caffeine, partly depending on prior usage. Caffeine is present in tea, coffee, chocolate, energy drinks (such as Red Bull), and some soft drinks, that in many people cause difficulty getting to sleep. Stage four, slow wave sleep, is reduced, and stage two sleep enhanced. These substances, therefore, should be avoided in the hours preceding going to bed. Withdrawal often leads to headaches and irritability.

Cocaine is a highly addictive stimulant that not only interferes with sleep, but may also cause strokes and heart attacks. Cocaine increases dopamine and serotonin in a part of the brain called the nucleus accumbens that is responsible for feelings of pleasure, and reward, which is why it is so addictive. Ingestion of cocaine increases wakefulness and suppresses REM sleep, which in turn affects memory. Withdrawal is reported to worsen the sleep disturbance, even though the person many believe that sleep is unchanged or improved. Cognitive performance is worse during withdrawal.

Nicotine is the second most often used stimulant. It increases vigilance and decreases sleeping time. Cigarette smoking is associated both with difficulty initiating and maintaining sleep, and with arousals on electroencephalograph recordings. Smoking promotes snoring and obstructive sleep apnea. Compared to nonsmokers, current smokers take longer to get to sleep, have less total sleep time, and have more stage one and less stage three and four sleep. Withdrawal from nicotine during sleep may be partly responsible for the shift towards lighter sleep. High prenatal smoking exposure modifies sleep patterns in premature babies by disrupting sleep organization and increasing nocturnal body movements.

Immune Function

Sleep and the immune system are closely linked. Infections alter sleep patterns and sleep patterns also affect the immune system. This interaction is dependant on the cytokine-immune-endocrine systems. Cytokines are signaling molecules that are produced by many cells in the body and are used to send messages between cells. Cytokines are critical to the development and functioning of the immune system. They are often produced by immune cells that have encountered an invading germ, thereby activating and recruiting further immune cells to increase the systems response to the invader. In the presence of infections there is an increase in sleepiness and lethargy. When an individual is sleep deprived there is an increased susceptibility to infection. Sleep deprivation leads to activation of the hypothalamic-pituitary-adrenal axis, with elevated glucocorticoid and cathecholamine plasma levels. A recent study by Sheldon Cohen et al. from Carnegie Mellon University in Pittsburgh, published in the *Archives of Internal Medicine* showed that healthy people who slept for less than seven hours a night were three times more likely to catch a cold than their more well-rested colleagues. They also reported that the quality of sleep was important, such that those who spent more time tossing and turning were more susceptible to catching a cold. This study involved 153 healthy volunteers who were kept in a hotel for five days after being infected with a cold virus. Another study showed that sleep deprivation caused a reduced antibody response to influenza vaccination compared to well-rested subjects.

From personal experience I know that sleep is altered during illness. In the acute phase of a systemic infection it can be very difficult to sleep, especially if there is a fever, but later in the illness, sleep may be enhanced. The peripheral immune system releases cytokines that react with receptors in the brain causing changes in physiological processes and complex behavior, including sleep. These changes collectively help the immune system to restore the individual to health. Cytokines also help to regulate sleep in the healthy state, some promoting sleep and others inhibiting sleep. Generally speaking a systemic infection will result in excessive sleepiness and fever, but with some infections sleep may be inhibited initially. There is some evidence that lack of sleep delays wound healing.

Exercise

It seems intuitive that regular vigorous physical activity would improve sleep, but there is surprisingly little research to confirm that that is indeed so. Certainly from my own observation I believe that I sleep much better when I have exercised vigorously during the day, and not so well if I have been sedentary. Compared to those who avoid exercise, physically fit people claim that they fall asleep more rapidly, sleep better and fee less tired during the day. These beliefs have been confirmed by studies that have demonstrated increased slow wave (deep sleep) in people who exercise regularly, compared to those who do not. King et al. studied physically inactive older adults, who were assigned to exercise or nonexercise groups for a period of sixteen weeks. The exercise group performed low-impact aerobics and brisk walking for 30 to 40 minutes four days week. At the end of the study the exercise group fell asleep in a shorter time, showed improved sleep quality, and slept longer than the nonexercise group. Another study of postmenopausal women showed that those who exercised at moderate intensity in the morning for three to four hours per week, were able to fall asleep more quickly than those exercising less.

The only caveat with exercise is that it is a stimulant, and therefore it is not advisable to exercise vigorously close to bedtime, however, a casual evening stroll is fine.

Sleep deprivation can affect exercise performance by reducing body temperature at rest, with a more rapid rise in body temperature during prolonged strenuous exercise, probably due to decreased sweating.

In a study from Indiana University, acute sleep deprivation reduced work time to exhaustion by an average of 11% and increased the perception of difficulty of the work. There was a very large variability in degree of impairment between individuals. Other studies have shown that sleep deprivation has had no effect on strength or speed.

Nutrition

There is accumulating evidence that lack of sleep may be a contributing factor to weight gain and obesity. The relationship between sleep and weight was first reported in the 1990s by researchers in Europe who were surprised to find that how much sleep a child got was a better predictor of being overweight than how much time was spent watching television. Watching television is often associated with snacking and when a person gets less sleep they have more time in which to eat, so one has to be careful in interpreting the data.

Subsequently the same relationship has been demonstrated in adults. In the Wisconsin Sleep Cohort Study, which tracks the sleep habits of nearly 3000 middle-aged government employees, those who reported sleeping less than eight hours per night were more likely to be overweight. These findings also need to be interpreted with caution, as overweight people are more likely to suffer from obstructive sleep apnea. Another study from Columbia University in New York City reported that there was a dose response relationship between sleeping time and incidence of obesity. Those sleeping six hours a night were 23% more likely to be obese than those sleeping between seven to nine hours per night. Those who slept five hours were 50% more likely, and those who slept four hours or less were 73% more likely to be obese.

There are two hormones that are affected by the quantity of sleep a person experiences, leptin and ghrelin. Leptin is released by fat cells and signals the brain to stop eating; ghrelin is released in the stomach and signals the brain to keep eating. Studies have shown that leptin levels are lower and ghrelin levels are higher in people who sleep fewer hours. In the Wisconsin Sleep Cohort Study, those who slept for five hours had 15% lower levels of leptin and 15% higher levels of ghrelin than those who slept for eight hours.

There is some evidence that sleep deprivation may do more than stimulate your appetite. Study done at the University of Chicago by Van Cauter et al. limited subjects to four hours of sleep for six consecutive nights. The results showed that they were 40% less able to clear glucose from their blood and 30% slower in releasing insulin than when they were allowed to sleep for twelve hours. This suggests that insulin sensitivity was decreased, which is the first step in developing type two diabetes.

There has been a dramatic increase in the incidence of obesity, type two diabetes and something called the metabolic syndrome, in the past few decades. The metabolic syndrome consists of a cluster of abnormalities, which include abdominal obesity, low HDL (good cholesterol), insulin resistance and elevated triglycerides, blood pressure and blood sugar. As we have seen, most if not all of these findings may be related to lack of sleep, and since sleep curtailment has become a very common practice in industrialized countries over the same period of time, one cannot help but think that there may be a connection.

Nocturia

Enlargement of the prostate gland is a very common condition in men as they get older and can be a significant cause of sleep disruption, as they have to get up several times each night to urinate (nocturia). The enlarging gland begins to obstruct the passageway out of the bladder, resulting in incomplete voiding, and therefore a shorter filling time. In addition the bladder becomes more sensitive causing a more frequent urge to void. Until recently the treatment was surgical in most cases, as the severity of the problem progressed, sometimes to complete obstruction. More recently effective medications have become available which can improve flow and actually shrink the gland, so that surgery is now much less common. There are two types of medication which each act in a different way to relieve the problem. The first type is a medication that relaxes the muscles in the prostate and bladder neck, improving flow and reducing symptoms. The second type lowers levels of a hormone (dihydrotestosterone) that is a major cause of prostate growth, but it may have to be taken for several months before improvement becomes apparent.

I have noticed that vigorous physical activity of at least one hour's duration through the day tends to reduce the frequency of having to urinate through the night. This is likely due to an increased secretion of antidiuretic hormone (ADH) (vasopressin) by the pituitary gland. Experimental data has shown that very vigorous and or prolonged moderately vigorous exercise increases the production and release of ADH by the pituitary gland. ADH helps to regulate fluid balance in the body by reducing the amount of urine production in the kidneys. Unfortunately as we get older the kidney becomes less responsive to the hormone, and therefore more urine is produced during the night. As mentioned earlier, obstructive sleep apnea also causes nocturia, which clears up with appropriate treatment of the sleep apnea.

Shift Work

Shift work is defined as a work schedule that is outside the typical 9-5 business day. Shift workers have been shown to be at increased risk for a variety of chronic illnesses such as cardiovascular and gastrointestinal diseases. Whether this is related to shift workers being awake and active through the night or because they tend to get fewer hours of sleep than traditional workers is unknown. Also shift workers have increased social stresses due to their work schedules.

The main complaints that shift workers present with

are insomnia, disrupted sleep schedules, reduced performance, difficulties with personal relationships, irritability and depressed mood.

Long distance drivers face some of the more serious challenges as they battle fatigue due to their irregular sleep schedules and long tedious hours on the road. Research shows that driver fatigue from sleep deprivation is one of the leading safety hazards in the transportation industry.

Other examples of shift workers are doctors, nurses, pilots, police officers, and fire fighters, all doing jobs that require alertness and quick decision making. The most serious problem that shift workers encounter as a result of their schedules is frequent sleep disturbance and associated excessive sleepiness while on the job. This in turn leads to poor concentration, absenteeism/presenteeism, accidents, errors, injuries and even fatalities. Examples of catastrophes in which fatigue from sleep deprivation has been thought to be a factor are Three Mile Island, the Exxon Valdez and the failure of the space shuttle Columbia.

Unfortunately shift work is necessary in modern life, so we need to learn how to make the best of an unavoidable situation. Swing shifts alternating two weeks of mornings and two weeks of evenings, that are prevalent on assembly lines in the automotive industry, are relatively easy to adjust to, as there is a core of five to six hours of sleep time with a two hour change from shift to shift. The more difficult shifts are intermittent and permanent night shifts.

Here are some suggestions for those working permanent night shifts. Wear dark glasses when driving home after the shift, keep the same bedtime and wake time even on weekends and days off (difficult to do from a social perspective), eliminate noise and light from the bedroom (use eye masks and ear plugs if necessary), avoid food and caffeinated beverages close to bedtime and avoid alcohol. Try to be exposed to us much bright light through the shift as possible, be physically active during breaks and drink a caffeinated beverage to help stay alert during the shift.

Some aircrews stay on their home base time, even if they are out of synch with everyone around them, and some sleep as they feel the need. Rest facilities are provided on long haul flights, so that aircrew can get some sleep on board the aircraft, and many long distance drivers have bunk beds in their cabs.

Recent research from Seattle is suggesting that women who work night shifts and who experience sleep deprivation, circadian disruption, and exposure to light at night are at increased risk of developing breast cancer and possibly colorectal cancer, due to altered nighttime melatonin levels and reproductive hormone profiles.

A recent review of twenty-two papers looking at associations between shift work and abortion, stillbirth, premature birth and birth weight, found no association between rotating shift work or fixed night shift and negative pregnancy outcomes. The authors did note some epidemiological support for a relationship between fixed night shift and late abortions/stillbirth, and recommended that pregnant women should avoid fixed night shifts.

Menopause

The literature on menopause and sleep is very mixed with some studies claiming no sleep disturbances due to menopause, and others linking hot flashes with sleep disturbances, even going so far as to suggest sleep disturbance in the presence of the hot flashes may be an indication for taking estrogen replacement.

It is apparent that women going through the menopause do have increased sleep disturbance compared to premenopausal women, but this could just be due to the physiology of ageing as opposed to being a symptom of menopause.

Jet Lag

Jet lag is a physiological condition that is a consequence of alterations to circadian rhythms, resulting from traveling across multiple time zones in a short time. Symptoms include, reduced alertness, nighttime insomnia, loss of appetite, depressed mood, poor psychomotor coordination and reduced cognitive skills.

Direction of travel makes a difference, with west to east being more difficult to adjust to than east to west, as it is easier to go to bed late than it is to get up early. The problem is of greater significance for airline personnel and business travelers than for holiday travelers, as they need to remain alert.

A number of strategies have been recommended to help prevent or overcome jet lag. Some people take melatonin to help reset the biological clock, others adjust their bedtime gradually for several days before traveling, and others just try to ignore the change. Several years ago I was traveling from Toronto, Canada, to London, England, on a regular basis for my work. The travel was overnight, arriving in England in the early morning. I have great difficulty trying to sleep on an airplane, so usually arrived having been awake all night. On arrival we took a taxi to the hospital and spent the morning getting our laboratory ready for work. After setting up the laboratory I would go for a jog and then have lunch, before starting work in the afternoon. After work I would stay up until my normal bedtime (local time).

Even though the literature fails to support vigorous physical activity helping to reset the biological clock, I found that if I jogged, I would be free from jet lag the next day, but if I did not then I would be less alert the following day.

Exposure to bright light also helps to rest the biological clock, by suppressing melatonin production at the time the person would normally be ready to sleep, so being exposed to outdoors light during the jog may have also been a factor.

Trying to sleep on an airplane can be something of a challenge, but one can try to remain hydrated by drinking water and avoiding alcohol and caffeinated beverages. Getting up and moving about the cabin on a regular basis is also beneficial. All these simple things help to reduce jet lag following the flight.

Restless Leg Syndrome

Restless leg syndrome is a condition characterized by an urge to move the arms and legs, coming on at rest, relieved by movement and worse in the evening or night than during the day. Sleep is disturbed by the movements of the limbs, not only for the sufferer, but also for the partner.

Endocrine System

Spiegel et al. from the University of Chicago published the results of a sleep deprivation study in the *Lancet,* which showed that sleep debt caused decreased glucose tolerance and TSH concentrations, and increased cortisol and sympathetic activity, compared to a nonsleep deprived state. They commented that the effects were similar to those seen with normal ageing.

The regulation of many hormones is dependent on the circadian rhythm and hence on sleep. Sleep deprivation has a profound effect on the endocrine system. In addition to the increase in cortisol production, there is a decrease in growth hormone release and a disturbance in autonomic tone. The autonomic nervous system refers to the sympathetic and parasympathetic nerves. With normal sleep the sympathetic nerve activity (tone) is decreased and the parasympathetic tone increased, but with sleep deprivation this is reversed. Most endocrine organs are very sensitive to changes in autonomic tone.

Behavioral (Sleep Hygiene and Lifestyle)

Sleep hygiene refers to how people approach sleeping and their behavior relating to preparing for sleep For instance many university students party late into the night or stay up all night preparing for an examination, and have little consistency with regard to a sleeping routine. The body has a circadian rhythm very close to twenty-four hours. In practice we generally work around a twenty-four hour clock and the body is adapted well to this periodicity.

The first point I want to make about sleep hygiene is that it is important to have a regular routine of going to bed at a constant time and getting up at a regular time. This is obviously not always possible, but the less deviation we have the better it is for our sleep. Going to bed late and getting up late on weekends is therefore not ideal. There are two times when we tend to get most drowsy, 2–4 A.M., and 2–4 P.M. taking naps through the day will often interfere with nocturnal sleep, and should therefore be avoided, or at least kept to a short duration. To avoid napping, it is good idea when feeling drowsy through the day to undertake some gentle exercise.

Avoid ingesting alcohol within two hours of going to bed, and avoid ingesting caffeine and or smoking tobacco within four hours of retiring. Gentle exercise such as a casual walk before bed is fine, but avoid strenuous physical activity within two hours of going to bed as it causes arousal and makes it difficult to get to sleep.

Tryptophan is an essential amino acid that is a precursor of serotonin and melatonin. An essential amino acid is a substance that the body cannot synthesize, and therefore must be ingested with our food. Some foods are rich in tryptophan and are therefore thought to promote sleep, although there is little good scientific evidence that they are effective. A study done in Australia, and published in 2007 in the *American Journal of Clinical Nutrition* showed that a high-glycemic-index carbohydrate meal consumed four hours before bedtime significantly shortened the time to fall asleep compared to subjects who ate low-glycemic-index meals. The glycemic index is a measure of how quickly the carbohydrate is absorbed into the blood after ingestion, a high index being faster than a low index. Carbohydrate intake is known to increase the plasma concentration of tryptophan. Therefore it is suggested that a snack consisting of crackers and a dairy product may be beneficial to sleep if consumed in the evening.

The bedroom should be as dark and as quiet as possible, and should be used only for sexual activity and sleeping. It is not a good idea to have a television in the room, or to take work to bed. A bedtime ritual of light reading prior to going to sleep may also be useful. The temperature of the room is also important, as it can be very disturbing to be too hot or cold.

Sleep is important to the proper functioning of the body.

Sleep disorders are common and under diagnosed.

Inadequate sleep is associated with coronary artery disease, strokes and obesity.

Sleep deprivation may be volitional or due to sleep disorders, and is associated with an increased incidence of accidents.

3
Eating

How much we eat is important, but I have always believed that what we eat is more important; after all we are the result of what we eat.

There are three main components of food: carbohydrates, fats, and proteins. All three are necessary for health, but the source, and balance between the groups, is crucial. The body utilizes these foods for growth, energy production, maintenance and repair.

Food is taken into the stomach and intestines where it is broken down into simpler forms, absorbed through the walls of the intestines, and carried by the blood to various organs and cells for storage or utilization. Much of the food is burned in the tissues to produce energy that allows us to be physically active, and to maintain and repair the body. Cells contain little furnaces called mitochondria, where food is burned and energy is produced. This process is known as metabolism, and in addition to producing energy, also produces water and carbon dioxide, which have to be eliminated from the body.

Each of the three food types produces different amounts of energy when burned. The amount of energy is quantified in kilocalories. One gram of carbohydrate when completely burned produces 4 kilocalories, one gram of protein 4 kilocalories and one gram of fat 9 kilocalories. Because one gram of fat has more kilocalories than a gram of carbohydrate or protein, fat is often referred to as calorie dense food. If one wanted to eat a lot of calories it would be easier to eat fat than protein or carbohydrate.

Under normal circumstances the body burns carbohydrate and fat in preference to protein. Protein is mostly utilized to manufacture and repair muscle. The brain can only use carbohydrate, and is very sensitive to blood glucose levels.

Carbohydrates

Carbohydrates may be classified as simple or complex. Simple carbohydrates are typically simple sugars of one sort or another, such as glucose, sucrose, lactose and fructose, whereas complex carbohydrates are three or more linked sugars. A good example of a simple carbohydrate would be a candy or can of regular pop, and a complex carbohydrate would be a fruit, vegetable or grain.

The digestive system breaks down ingested carbohydrates into simple sugar molecules (mostly glucose), small enough to be transported into the blood stream. Some carbohydrates are better for you than others. In general easily digested carbohydrates from white bread, white rice, pastries, pop and other highly processed foods are less healthy than carbohydrates obtained from whole grains, beans, fruits and vegetables.

They glycemic index (GI) describes how quickly and how high an ingested carbohydrate raises the blood sugar compared to pure glucose (100). David Jenkins developed the concept at the University of Toronto in 1980, in order to improve the diets of diabetic patients. Carbohydrates can be divided into low GI <55, medium GI 56 to 69 and high >70.

In general, oats, barley, bran, whole grain breads, brown rice, pasta, noodles, fruits and vegetables are considered to have low GI. For a comprehensive list of the GI of foods, go to the Web site www.glycemicindex.com at the University of Sidney in Australia, which lists over 1200 foods.

A diet consisting of mainly low GI foods will avoid fluctuations of blood glucose and insulin secretion, with less stress on the homeostatic systems. It also delays the feeling of hunger between meals.

One criticism of the GI is that you can have a food that has very little carbohydrate, but a high GI, compared to a food with a lot of carbohydrate and a low GI. To address this issue researchers have developed the concept of glycemic load (GL). GL is calculated by multiplying the GI by the amount of carbohydrate contained in the food. A GL of >20 is considered to be high, 11 to 19 medium and <10 low.

The way a food is processed can alter the GI and GL; for example pure unadulterated apple juice has a GI of 39 and a GL of 9.6, whereas the raw apple has a GI of 39, but a GL of 5.7.

The general consensus of the various expert bodies on diet seems to be that carbohydrates should provide between 45 and 65% of our calorie intake. Highly active people such as competitive athletes probably need to be at the high end of the range. We should try to have the majority of our intake in the form of complex carbohydrates and minimize our simple carbohydrate intake, unless we need a rapid supply of glucose. A situation requiring a rapid glucose intake might be an athlete in competition requiring a quick energy source, or an insulin reaction in a diabetic, when the blood sugar falls to a dangerously low level and interferes with brain function.

Grains are the seeds of grasses. They are commonly harvested and used as food for both humans and cattle. The most common are barley, bulgur, cracked wheat, oats, rice and whole wheat. Flax is sometimes lumped in as a grain as it has many of the same nutrients, plus some important additional ones.

They may be marketed as whole grains or as processed grains (brown bread versus white bread). Whole grains contain all three of the components that make up the seed, the husk, germ, and endosperm, and have greater food and health value than processed grains, which are missing the husk.

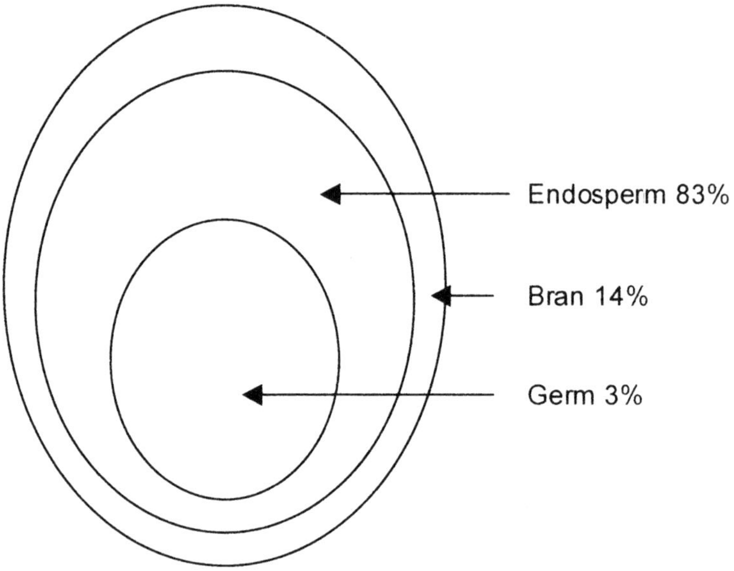

Figure 3. Cross section of grain

Whole grains are a good source of fiber, minerals and vitamins. Oats and flax have some special and different properties than the others.

Oats have a relatively high fat content for a grain and contain a soluble fiber called beta glucan. Beta glucan is responsible for a decrease and delay in the rise of blood sugar following a meal in type 2 diabetes, and also helps to lower the level of LDL, the so called bad cholesterol, in the blood.

Flax seed also has a high fat content, containing high levels of alpha linoleic acid, an omega 3 fatty acid, and fiber. Flax seed has a tough outer coat and unless it is milled, to break the outer coat, will pass through the intestine unchanged, and without nutritional benefit. It also helps to slow and reduce the rise in blood sugar following a meal, and may also help to lower LDL.

Fruits and vegetables are an important source of complex carbohydrates, vitamins, insoluble fiber, minerals and phytochemicals. The mothers of the world have long urged their offspring to eat their fruits and vegetables in order to be healthy, and science has now proved them to be correct.

Current dietary recommendations suggest that we should have a minimum intake of five, and up to thirteen servings of fruits and vegetables (2½ to 6½ cups) per day, depending on the total calorie intake required. For example, a person eating 2000 calories per day should have nine servings of fruit and vegetables. Canada's food guide says five to ten servings per day.

There is a great deal of evidence to indicate that a diet rich in fruits and vegetables is associated with a lower risk of coronary artery disease and stroke. A very large study from the Nurses Health Study and the Health Professionals Follow-up Study, looked at the dietary habits and health of almost 110,000 men and women. The results indicated that those who ate eight or more servings of fruit and vegetables a day, compared to those who ate less than 1½ servings a day, were 30% less likely to have a heart attack or stroke.

A meta analysis of these and other long-term studies

done in the United States and Europe, reported similar results. Those who ate more than five servings of fruit and vegetables a day were 20% less likely to have coronary artery disease and a stroke than those who ate less than three servings a day.

Diet can also influence blood pressure. The DASH study reported in 1997 in *The New England Journal of Medicine* showed a significant lowering of blood pressure as a result of changes in diet. DASH stands for Dietary Approaches to Stop Hypertension. The DASH diet required a high intake of fruits, vegetables, and low fat dairy foods, with a low intake of saturated fat, total fat and cholesterol. Those subjects on the DASH diet reduced their systolic and diastolic blood pressure by 5.5 and 3.0 mm Hg respectively compared to controls, but those subjects who had systolic pressures greater than 140 and diastolic pressures greater than 90 mm Hg reduced their systolic and diastolic blood pressures by 11.4 and 5.5 mm Hg. In other words the benefit was even greater if you already had high blood pressure before you started the diet.

Although all fruits and vegetables are probably beneficial, green leafy vegetables such as romaine lettuce, kale, bok choi and spinach; cruciferous vegetables such as broccoli and cabbage; and citrus fruits such as oranges and grapefruit are likely the most beneficial. There are numerous studies that indicate that a diet rich in fruits and vegetables may be protective against some forms of cancer, but there are other studies that show no benefit. A report from the World Cancer Research Fund and the American Institute for Cancer research published in 2007, suggests that vegetables such as lettuce, broccoli, bok choi, cabbage and onions, as well as fruits, may protect against cancers of the gastrointestinal tract, and lungs.

There is also some evidence to suggest that tomatoes

and tomato-based products may afford some protection from prostate cancer, perhaps due to a chemical responsible for their red color (lyocopene). Lycopene is one of a group of chemicals called carotenoids that the body is able to turn into vitamin A. Carotenoids are found in brightly colored fruits and vegetables.

Another fruit that has recently been found to have beneficial effects for prostate cancer is pomegranate. Pomegranate juice has antioxidant properties thought to be due to ellagic acid, which slows the growth of, and causes cancer cells to self-destruct, a process known as apoptosis.

Intake of fruits and vegetables is important for eyesight; in particular for the prevention of cataracts and macular degeneration, two conditions associated with ageing. These conditions are accelerated by the production of free radicals, generated by exposure to ultra violet radiation (sunlight), cigarette smoke, air pollution, infections and metabolism. Free radicals are highly reactive particles that damage cell walls unless they are mopped up by the body's defense system first. They are a by-product of metabolism, and in its defense, the body produces antioxidants that convert free radicals to harmless particles. We also obtain antioxidants from our food; two of these, lutein and zeaxanthin, are found in dark green leafy vegetables such as spinach and kale. These two antioxidants accumulate in the eyes and help to protect the tissues of the eyes from free radicals and the damage that results.

Cherries and blueberries are two fruits that have a very high antioxidant content. Red grapes contain an antioxidant called resveratrol that may account for some of the health benefit attributed to red wine, however that benefit can also be obtained by drinking red grape juice if you wish to avoid alcohol. The many and varied antioxidants contained in fruits and vegetables are thought to be a major reason for their observed health benefits.

Fats

There are basically four types of fat, polyunsaturated, monounsaturated, saturated and trans fat. Fats are made up of chains of carbon atoms with hydrogen ions attached and a carboxyl group at the end of the chain (COOH). Each

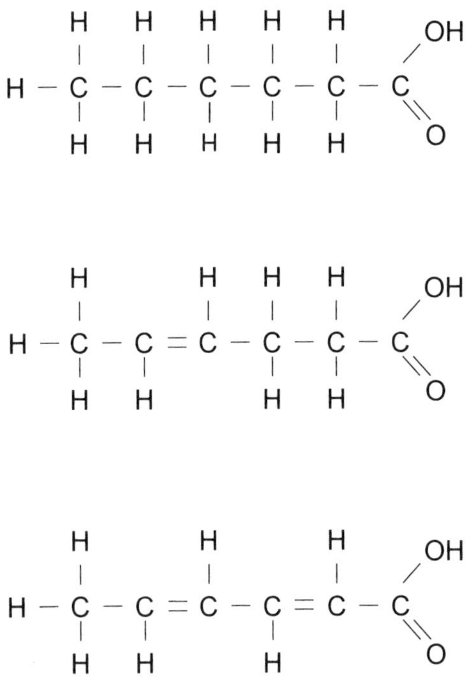

Saturated

Mono Unsaturated

Poly Unsaturated

Figure 4. Structure of fats with bond

carbon atom has four bonds (hooks) and can attach to four other atoms, oxygen has two and hydrogen has one. When one of the carbon hooks is not attached to a hydrogen atom, the hook connects to the adjacent carbon to form a double bond.

Polyunsaturated fats have more than one double bond, monounsaturated fats have one double bond and saturated fats have no double bonds. Double bonds affect the shape and properties of the fat molecules, the more saturated the fat, the more solid the fat. The less saturated the fat, the more liquid the fat, hence butter, a saturated fat, is solid at room temperature, whereas olive oil a monounsaturated fat is liquid at room temperature. The reason for this is that saturated fat chains are straight, whereas unsaturated fat chains are bent and therefore cannot be packed together as tightly as saturated chains. Think of the chains as being wooden matchsticks in a matchbox. As long as the matchsticks are straight they will all fit into the box, but if we empty them out and bend all of the matchsticks, we will no longer be able to fit them all back into the box.

Unsaturated fats tend to be liquid at room temperature and have a short shelf life before becoming rancid. Double bonds are less stable than single bonds, and therefore unsaturated fats are subject to picking up hydrogen atoms. For this reason manufacturers use a process called hydrogenation, during which hydrogen is bubbled through the fat to partially saturate it, thereby making it more solid and spreadable, as well as giving it a longer shelf life. Unfortunately this process turns good fat into bad fat, producing trans fat that behaves like a saturated fat, even though it is monounsaturated, and it is thought to be the unhealthiest form of fat.

Unsaturated fat comes in two forms, cis and trans. The cis form has the two hydrogens missing on the same side of the chain, and is as a result bent. The trans fat has one hydrogen missing on either side of the chain and is therefore

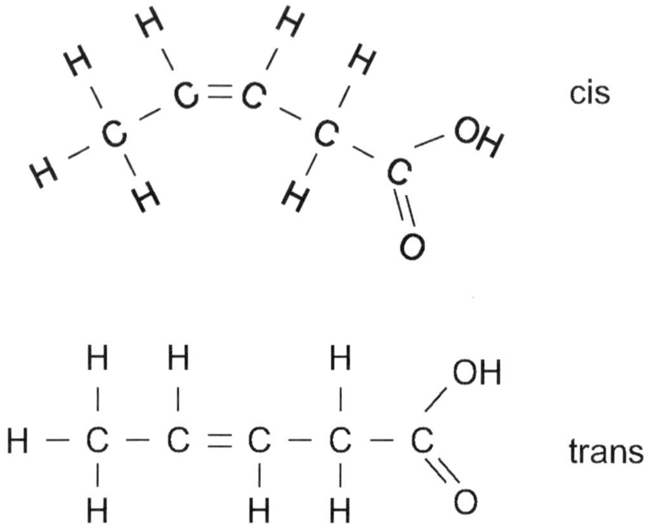

Figure 5. Diagram of cis and trans

straight, which is why it behaves as a saturated fat.

As a general rule animal fats are saturated and vegetable fats are unsaturated. Excessive amounts of saturated fats are bad for health and are associated with high cholesterol levels and an increased incidence of cardiovascular disease, whereas mono and poly unsaturated fats are healthier.

The bad publicity that fat has received has led to the mistaken idea that all fat is bad. Fat is an essential part of our diet and is necessary for health; it is the type and amount that is critical. Another misconception is that a person has to have a high cholesterol intake in order to have a high blood level. Fat (especially saturated fat), is converted into cholesterol in the body, so it is not necessary to have a high cholesterol intake in order to have high blood cholesterol. All cells contain cholesterol in their walls and therefore it is a vital substance for our health.

The current recommendation is that less than 30% of our total calorie intake should come from fat, less than 7% should be in the form of saturated fat and less than 1% trans fat. This means that we have to limit our intake of animal fat and processed foods. Many processed foods such as cookies and baked goods contain hydrogenated fats, which in turn means that they have a high trans fat content. No amount of trans fat is considered to be safe, even though it appears in small quantities in naturally occurring foods. Trans fat has been shown to increase the levels of bad cholesterol (LDL) while at the same time decreasing the levels of good cholesterol (HDL). These changes are associated with an increased risk of coronary artery disease and heart attacks. The Canadian government has a task force that has established limits for trans fats and is monitoring their presence in foods. The limit for vegetable oil and margarine is 2% of total fat, and for all other foods is 5% of total fat.

The majority of our fat intake should come from vegetable oils, low fat dairy products, fish, lean meat, poultry, fruits and nuts.

Omega 6 and omega 3 fats are known as essential fatty acids, because they cannot be manufactured in the body, and are important building blocks for many compounds required to keep the body healthy.

Omega 3 fatty acids include alpha linolenic acid (ALA), eicosapentaenoic acid (EPA), and docosahexaenoic acid (DHA), all of which are polyunsaturated. They all have a double bond in the third carbon from the end of the chain, which is why they are called omega 3 fatty acids.

Omega 6 fatty acid is called linoleic acid and has a double bond in the carbon that is sixth from the end of the chain.

The products derived from omega 3 and omega 6 fatty acids have opposing effects in the body, but are all essential to our well being. Omega 3 products tend to be anti-inflammatory and omega 6 products tend to be inflammatory. They therefore play a role in our immune defense system.

Omega 3 and 6 fatty acids are found in the highest quantities in grains, seeds, nuts and fatty fish. Omega 3 has been shown to significantly reduce the chances of having a heart attack or stroke, and has also been shown to reduce the incidence of sudden death from heart rhythm disturbances. The GISSI-Prevenzione trial published in *The Lancet* in 1999, studied patients who had had a recent heart attack, over a three and a half year period, and found that those who took 1 gram per day of omega 3 fatty acids had 20% reduction in all cause deaths, a 30% reduction in cardiovascular deaths and a 45% reduction in sudden cardiac deaths. This is the reason why it is currently recommended to eat fish at least twice a week, and why some doctors are now prescribing fish oil for their heart patients.

Fish oil supplements have been shown to increase the breakdown of fibrin (a compound involved in clot and scar formation), to reduce blood pressure, and to reduce blood triglyceride levels. Other studies have found benefits in patients with rheumatoid arthritis. High doses of fish oil may be associated with an increased risk of bleeding. Doses of up to 3 grams of total EPA/DHA are considered to be safe.

There is some concern about mercury contamination of fish. Fish that are predatory, and longer lived are more likely to accumulate mercury than their smaller shorter-lived brethren. Health Canada suggests that it is safe to eat the following fish freely. Anchovy, Capelin, Char, Hake, Herring, Sardines, Atlantic mackerel, Mullet, Pollock, Salmon, Smelt, Sole, Rainbow Trout, Lake Whitefish, Blue Crab, Shrimp, Mussel, and Oyster. The provincial health services authority of British Columbia published an information bulletin in April 2008 that can be found in the Internet, with specific recommendations for type and amount of fish consumption for various age groups.

Several studies have reported possible anti-cancer effects of omega 3 fatty acids for breast, colon and prostate cancers, but the evidence is somewhat tenuous, and the jury is still out.

A recent article published in *The Canadian Medical Association Journal* by David Jenkins et al., questions the validity of recommending increased fish consumption, based on evidence that the present rate of harvesting does not appear to be sustainable. Scientists have projected that if present trends continue there will be a collapse of all commercially exploited fish stocks by mid century. It would seem prudent therefore to look for alternative sources of omega 3 fatty acids.

Cholesterol is an essential component of cell membranes where it is responsible for membrane permeability and fluidity. High levels in the blood are associated with atherosclerosis, a condition that is characterized by the plugging up of the blood vessels, by the formation of fatty plaques in the walls of the arteries, causing a decrease in the flow of blood.

The name cholesterol is derived from the Greek chole (bile), steros solid), and the chemical suffix –ol for an alcohol. Francois Poulletier de la Salle first identified it in 1769 in solid form, in gallstones.

Some cholesterol is ingested in the diet, but the majority (about 1 gram per day) is synthesized in the body from dietary fat, primarily in the liver.

Cholesterol is insoluble in blood and in order to be transported in the blood, has to be combined with protein to form lipoproteins. There is a large range of lipoprotein particles in blood, varying from very large to very small. The largest are called chylomicrons and give plasma a milky appearance. In descending order of size the others are, very low-density lipoproteins (VLDL), intermediate-density lipoproteins (IDL) low-density lipoproteins (LDL), and high-density lipoproteins (HDL). VLDL would be like a large whiffle ball, and HDL would be like a billiard ball.

The various forms of low-density lipoproteins are taken up by the cells and used in the tissues. Excess amounts of LDL are transported back to the liver where they are processed and secreted in bile. LDL is the lipoprotein that has been associated with clogging up the arteries and that is why it is often called bad cholesterol. HDL removes excess LDL from the blood, transporting it to the liver, and is therefore called good cholesterol. Think of excess LDL as a accumulating garbage, and HDL as garbage trucks. The major dietary sources of cholesterol are cheese, egg yolk, beef, pork, poultry, squid and shrimp. Plant based food sources do not contain cholesterol, but may contain cholesterol-like compounds called phytosterols, that actually help to lower cholesterol levels in the blood.

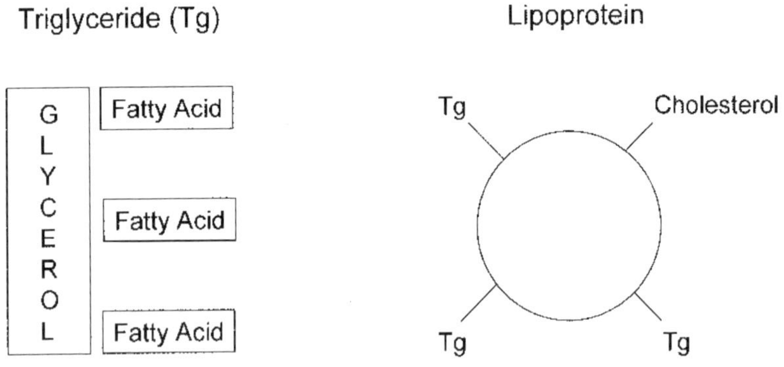

Figure 6. Diagrams of triglyceride and lipoprotein

The recommended cholesterol intake is less than 300 mg per day. One egg yolk contains 264 mg of cholesterol, and is a common constituent of baked goods.

Triglyceride consists of glycerol with three fatty acids attached, and is a major component of chylomicrons and VLDL. It is insoluble unless attached to protein as lipoprotein.

Triglycerides are split off in the tissues and used for energy production. Fat cells and liver cells can synthesize and store triglycerides. When the body requires fatty acids for energy production, the hormone glucagon initiates the breakdown of triglycerides by lipase, into fatty acids. The glycerol component can be converted into glucose.

High levels of triglycerides in the blood have been linked to atherosclerosis. There is a strong inverse relation between triglyceride level and HDL cholesterol level. There are different numbers recommended for total cholesterol and LDL levels in the blood, depending on the degree of risk that an individual has for developing heart disease. For healthy low risk individuals it is recommended that total cholesterol should be below 6.2 mmol/L, and LDL blood level should be below 3.4 mmol/L. HDL levels should be above 1mmol/L and the higher the better, as it seems to have a protective effect. Triglyceride blood level is recommended to be below 1.7 mmol/L. Different numbers are recommended for those who already have coronary artery disease and or are at increased risk of developing it. These numbers change from time to time depending on research results, so if this applies to you, you need to check with your doctor.

Diet is a very important means of controlling cholesterol levels in the body, but endurance aerobic exercise is a very effective way to increase HDL levels, and decrease triglyceride levels. Smoking cigarettes is a very effective way of decreasing HDL levels which is another good reason for not doing it.

Proteins

Proteins are organic compounds consisting of amino acids. There are twenty amino acids used in protein synthesis within the body, nine of which are called essential, because the body cannot make them and requires that they be ingested in food. Proteins participate in every process within cells. Many are enzymes that are needed for biochemical processes and are vital to metabolism. Some proteins also have structural and mechanical functions, such as actin and myosin, that make our muscles work. Others have varied functions such as forming scaffolding that maintains cell shape, taking part in cell signaling, and enabling immune responses. Protein is used for building, maintaining and repairing muscle, skin, blood and other tissues Very little protein is used as fuel when calorie supply is adequate, but in cases where energy supply is deficient, as in starvation, protein is converted to carbohydrate by a process known as gluconoegenesis to provide energy. Energy production takes priority over tissue building.

Dietary sources of protein include meats, fish, eggs, nuts, grains, legumes, and dairy products such as milk and cheese. Some sources such as milk, eggs, meat, and soy protein contain all the essential amino acids and are known as complete proteins, thereby having the most value to the body.

The best vegetable sources of protein are the pulses. Pulses are the edible seeds of legumes, like lentils, beans, peas and chickpeas. Pulses are unique in the plant kingdom in their ability to take nitrogen from the air and with the help of certain soil bacteria, turn it into a form that can be used by plants.

Lentils contain high levels of protein, and all but two of the essential amino acids. They are also a good source of fiber, vitamins and minerals, especially iron. Canada is the largest export producer of lentils in the world, but India is the largest producer. Chickpea (garbanzo beans) are high in protein and fiber, and also contain a lot of calcium and iron, along with vitamins and other minerals.

By combining plant food proteins it is possible to get all the essential amino acids. There are four groups of plant foods that contain proteins: group 1, breads, cereals and grains: group 2, legumes; group 3, vegetables; and group 4, nuts and seeds. By combining food from group 1, with food from any of the other three groups one can obtain all the essential amino acids.

Biological value (BV) is a measure of the proportion of absorbed protein from a food that is incorporated into the proteins of the body. Different protein sources have different levels of BV. The BV of plant protein is in general lower than that of animal protein. The standard for BV is egg white with a value of 100, which means that most of the absorbed nitrogen from egg white protein can be retained and used by the body. The BV of corn for example is 70, and peanut is 40, considerably less than the BV of egg white. About 15% of total calorie intake should come from protein, with some variation depending on the level and type of physical activity. Another way of calculating daily protein requirements recommends an intake of 0.8 grams of protein per kilogram of lean body weight, with an increase to 1-1.4 grams per kilogram of lean body weight for athletes.

If excess protein is consumed, it is converted in the body to sugars or fatty acids. This process releases nitrogen that is incorporated into urea that in turn is excreted by the kidney. Sometimes the kidney is overworked in this situation, and protein intake must then be restricted. Protein requirements are increased after injury, surgery, or after periods of starvation.

Specific proteins may be the cause of allergies, and allergic reaction to foods. The most common are casein in milk, gluten in wheat, proteins in peanuts, and shellfish. Animal and vegetable proteins likely have the same effects on health, but the package they come in can make a big difference. For example a 6-ounce steak is a very good source of protein providing 38 grams, along with 36 grams of fat, 13 grams of which is saturated. The same amount of salmon delivers 34 grams of protein, 18 grams of fat of which 4 grams is saturated. A cup of cooked lentils provide 18 grams of protein, but only 1 gram of fat. The lesson then, is that one needs to pay attention to what comes along with the protein. It is prudent to pick fish, poultry, whole grains, legumes, and low fat dairy products whenever possible.

Fiber

Fiber includes all the parts of plant foods that the body cannot digest or absorb, commonly called roughage. It passes through the stomach and bowel largely unchanged. It is found in varying quantities in fruits, vegetables, whole grains and legumes. It has the ability to prevent or relieve constipation as well as lowering the risk of diabetes and heart disease. There are two types of fiber, soluble and insoluble, which have different actions in the bowel.

Soluble fiber dissolves in water to form a gel-like material that can help to lower blood cholesterol and blood sugar levels. Examples of foods that have a large quantity of soluble fiber are oats, peas, beans, apples, citrus fruits, carrots, barley and psyllium, and they have a low glycemic index. Psyllium is the main ingredient in Metamucil that is used to prevent and treat constipation.

Insoluble fiber promotes the movement of material through the digestive system, and increases stool bulk. It is found in whole wheat flour, wheat bran, nuts and many vegetables.

A diet that is high in fiber helps to promote regular bowel movements and prevent hemorrhoids and diverticulosis. It may also be beneficial to those people who have irritable bowel syndrome.

The suggested fiber intake for healthy males is 38 grams per day for those under fifty years of age and 30 grams per day for those over fifty. For women it is 25 grams per day under fifty and 21 grams per day over fifty years of age. The average North American dietary intake of fiber is about 15 grams per day.

Many people find that high fiber dietary intake is associated with increased gas production and are therefore reluctant to increase their intake of fiber. Over time this problem seems to settle if one perseveres, and in any case the benefits far outweigh the inconvenience and or embarrassment.

Alcohol

Alcohol comes in three major categories, wine, beer and spirits. The category is important in determining what comes with the alcohol. Wine, particularly red wine, comes with antioxidants. Beer comes with yeast and vitamins, but spirits come with no food value other than calories. These calories are therefore called empty calories. There is good evidence that small quantities of alcohol, especially wine, may be beneficial to health. There is a decreased mortality rate amongst those who have one or two standard drinks per day (4 oz of wine, 350 ml of beer or 1 oz of spirits) compared to those that have none, or those who have more. Small amounts of alcohol have also been shown to increase the level of HDL in the blood.

In spite of these findings it is not recommended that people who do not presently drink alcoholic beverages should start to do so, but it is recommended that those who drink more than the suggested amounts should decrease their intake.

Excessive amounts of alcohol intake are associated with an increase in the risk of accidental injury to self and others, liver disease (cirrhosis), inflammation of the pancreas, brain damage, and social and work problems.

Vitamins

Vitamins are organic compounds required by the body that cannot be manufactured in sufficient quantity by the body, and therefore must be obtained from the diet. There are thirteen vitamins in all, and these may be divided into two groups, fat-soluble and water-soluble. The fat-soluble vitamins are vitamins A, D, E and K. the water-soluble vitamins are the eight B vitamins and vitamin C, and are not readily stored in the body, resulting in the need for regular intake in food. Fat-soluble vitamins by virtue of being fat soluble, are readily stored in the body, which can lead to toxicity from excessive intake. Vitamins serve many different biochemical functions, including acting as hormones, antioxidants, mediators of cell signaling, regulators of cell and tissue growth and differentiation. They also act as catalysts in metabolism, and may have anticancer properties.

The history of vitamins is very interesting. Apparently Hippocrates discovered that eating liver cured night blindness, which we now know to be a condition caused by vitamin A deficiency.

In 1747, James Lind a British Royal naval surgeon, carried out one of the first clinical trials in medical history and discovered that the ingestion of citrus fruits helped to prevent scurvy, and could actually cure the condition. This was a very important discovery as many sailors became sick and died during long voyages as a result of the disease. In fact it is estimated that the British navy lost more sailors from scurvy than they did from battles at sea. As a result of Lind's discovery the navy eventually supplied their sailors with citrus fruits, and that is why the British sailors became known as limeys. We now know that the cause of scurvy is a deficiency of vitamin C.

During the Second World War, Allied prisoners in Japanese prison camps were fed a diet of white rice, and many developed a condition known as beriberi, due to a deficiency of vitamin B1 (thiamin). The irony of this is that it was a British-trained Japanese naval medical doctor, Takaki Kanehiro, who first observed in 1884 that a diet of white rice was associated with the development of beriberi. Thiamin is present in rice bran and that is why brown rice should replace white rice in the diet.

The following is a list of vitamins with their major dietary sources followed by the conditions that result from deficiencies of the vitamins.

Vitamin A (Retinol/Beta Carotene) Present in fish, shrimp, milk, butter, eggs, spinach, broccoli, endive and orange vegetables. Deficiency causes night blindness and keratomalacia (dry eyes).

Vitamin B1 (Thiamin) Present in wheat germ, whole

grains, beef and pork, organ meats, rice bran, soybeans, peanuts and nuts. Deficiency causes beriberi, a condition that can affect the nervous system and the heart, in severe cases leading to heart failure and death.

Vitamin B2 (Riboflavin) Present in organ meats, beef and pork, chicken, milk cheese, eggs, spinach and yeast. Deficiency causes ariboflavinosis that is manifest by cracking at the sides of the mouth.

Vitamin B3 (Niacin) Present in beef, liver, turkey, tuna, salmon, milk, eggs, legumes, whole grains, peanuts and yeast. Deficiency causes pellagra, a condition that is characterized by diarrhea, dermatitis, dementia and death.

Vitamin B6 (Pantothenic acid) Present in lobster, eggs, cheese, corn, peas, soybeans, sunflower seeds and yeast. Deficiency causes paresthesia, the medical term for the feeling of 'pins and needles'.

Vitamin B6 (Pyridoxine) Present in beef and pork, fish, eggs, whole grains, carrots, sunflower seeds and yeast. Deficiency causes anemia, the medical term for insufficient hemoglobin in the blood.

Vitamin B7 (Biotin) Present in liver, butter, eggs, rice, peas, soybeans, sunflower seeds and yeast. Deficiency causes dermatitis and enteritis (inflammation of the skin and bowel).

Vitamin B9 (Folic acid) Present in liver, barley, leafy green vegetables, soybeans, beans, lentils and yeast.

Deficiency during pregnancy is a cause of birth defects such as spina bifida, otherwise anemia with larger than normal red blood cells.

Vitamin B12 (Cyancobalamin) Present in beef, liver, fish, eggs and cheese. Deficiency causes a particular type of anemia, (where the red blood cells are larger than normal), and degeneration of part of the spinal cord.

Vitamin C (Ascorbic acid) Present in rose hips, broccoli, brussel sprouts, spinach, green peppers, citrus fruits and black currants. Deficiency causes scurvy that is manifest by skin sores, rash, break down of previous wounds, swollen and bleeding gums with loss of teeth and muscle weakness.

Vitamin D (Cholecalciferol) Present in liver, fish, cod liver oil, margarine, eggs, and mushroom. Most milk has vitamin D added. Also synthesized in the skin with exposure to ultraviolet rays from the sun. Deficiency is the cause of Rickets and Osteomalacia, conditions manifest by impaired bone formation.

More recent work suggests that vitamin D may be important in preventing cancer, and those of us who live at northern or southern latitudes may require supplementation, especially in the fall and winter months. Vitamin D is synthesized in the skin in response to exposure to ultraviolet radiation from the sun, as well as being ingested with our food. Because exposure to ultraviolet radiation is associated with the development of skin cancer, we are advised to use sun block and cover our skin so as to avoid being exposed. This reduces the amount of vitamin D being produced in the skin, and while it may not be sufficient to cause deficiency symptoms, it may be enough to reduce the blood level to an amount that is suboptimal.

Calcium and vitamin D supplements are routinely advised for post menopausal women to help prevent osteoporosis. Scientists have observed that those women taking supplements had a much higher blood level of vitamin D than those that did not take supplements. What was startling was that after three years, the women who had the high blood levels of vitamin D had 60% less cancer than those with lower blood levels. As a result of this study, published in the *American Journal of Nutrition,* the cancer society is recommending that people living in Canada should take a supplement of 1000 IU of vitamin D daily during the fall and winter months. Adults at higher risk of having lower vitamin D levels should consider taking vitamin D supplementation all year round. This includes people who are older, have dark skin, and who don't go outside often, or who wear clothing that cover most of their skin. The previous recommendation was to take 200 to 600 IU daily depending on age.

Vitamin E (Tocopherol) Present in wheat germ, plant oils, margarine, cabbage, sunflower seeds and nuts. Deficiency is somewhat controversial in humans. There has been a lot of research into vitamin E because it is a powerful antioxidant and there are good reasons as to why it should be beneficial in protecting against heart disease. Research has produced mixed findings. The consensus presently is that there is no demonstrable benefit to taking vitamin E supplements. This may be in part, because there are eight different forms of the vitamin, each with different biological potency.

Vitamin K (Phyonadione) Present in liver, oats, cheese and green vegetables. Deficiency results in a tendency to bleed easily.

Health Canada has published Canada's food guide, giving recommended dietary intakes for all the food groups, vitamins and minerals. The National Academy of Sciences Institute of Medicine and Nutrition Board has published dietary reference intakes (DRIs), which replace the old recommended nutrient intakes (RNIs).

One subset of the DRIs is the recommended dietary allowance (RDA). The RDA is the average daily intake of a nutrient that is sufficient to meet the requirement of nearly all (97–98%) healthy persons.

The RDA is the amount of a nutrient required to prevent deficiency diseases, and not necessarily the amount required for optimal health.

Minerals

There are six major minerals and then trace minerals for which we have RDAs.

Calcium is found in carob, dairy products, sardines, sesame seeds and nuts. Many foods such as some brands of orange juice are now fortified with calcium, and some commonly used over-the-counter medications such as Tums contain large quantities of calcium. Deficiency is associated with the loss of bone mass and strength (osteoporosis), seizures and muscle spasms.

Iodine is present in seafood, seaweed and milk. All table salt in Canada is fortified with iodine. Deficiency causes cretinism in children and goiters in adults.

Iron is found in liver, beef, egg yolks, nuts, seafood, and seaweed and whole gains. Deficiency is a major cause of anemia.

Magnesium is found in molasses, nuts, fish and whole grains. Deficiency can cause tremors, muscle spasms, confusion, delirium and seizures.

Phosphorous is present in fish, meat and dairy products. Deficiency is very rare but when it does occur, results in bone pain and brittle bones with weakness and loss of appetite.

Zinc is found in liver, meat, eggs, seafood and whole grains. Deficiency causes diarrhea, loss of appetite and hair loss.

Trace minerals are chromium, copper, fluoride, manganese, molybdenum, potassium, selenium and sodium. Only two of these, potassium and sodium, are commonly associated with problems related to having too little or too much.

The blood levels of potassium and sodium are most often out of the normal range as a result of medications taken for medical illnesses. Low blood potassium levels are associated with muscle weakness, muscle cramps and spasms, and heart rhythm disturbances. High blood potassium levels cause abnormal heart rhythms and eventually stop the heart from beating.

Potassium is found in citrus fruits, bananas, tomatoes, beef, potatoes and raisins. Low blood sodium levels cause muscle cramps, stomach cramps, nausea and fatigue. High blood sodium levels increase blood pressure and water retention. Sodium usually come as salt in the diet. Processed food and canned soups are particularly high in sodium, but it is also present in snack foods, margarine, sardines, milk, cabbage and bread. Most people add salt in their cooking, and also have a saltshaker on the table thus adding to an already greater than required salt load.

Research has shown that salt restriction in the diet is associated with lower blood pressures, and has suggested that a modest reduction of salt added to processed foods, would significantly reduce the number of people having to be treated with medication for high blood pressure.

A salt restricted diet has also been found to be beneficial in those people with asthma, reducing symptoms and improving function.

The main sources of sodium in the average North American diet are, 77% from processed foods, 12% from natural sources, 6% added to food while eating and 5% added during cooking. Recommended sodium intake for healthy people varies from 1000 mg to 1500 mg per day depending on age.

StatsCan recently released data indicating that Canadian men consumed an average of 4100 mg of sodium daily while women consumed 2900 mg.

In general, people should seek foods that have high potassium content, and avoid foods with high sodium content. High intakes of potassium and calcium are associated with lower blood pressures.

A good example of the importance of sodium in relationship to blood pressure is the DASH-sodium trial. The DASH-sodium diet was like the DASH diet, but additionally reduced sodium intake, and was associated with a much greater drop in blood pressure than that seen with DASH alone.

Supplements

Conventional wisdom says that a balanced diet, rich in fruits and vegetables, provides all of the required nutrients for a healthy individual. However, there are certain situations in which dietary supplementation is undoubtedly helpful. Calcium and vitamin D supplementation for people with osteopenia and osteoporosis is prescribed routinely, and now the cancer society is calling for vitamin D supplementation in the fall and winter months for Canadians.

There is a condition where the stomach no longer secretes acid, which prevents the absorption of vitamin B12 from food, leading to anemia. Vitamin B12 must be injected to prevent or cure the anemia.

Breakfast cereals are fortified with vitamin B, and all cow's milk is fortified with vitamin D. Bread is fortified with folic acid and pregnant women are usually advised to take extra folic acid and iron. Folic acid supplementation during pregnancy has been shown to reduce the incidence of a congenital abnormality of the nervous system known as neural tube defect in babies.

There is some evidence that supplementation with vitamin C shortens the duration of upper respiratory symptoms in colds.

There are other conditions such as food allergies or restricted calorie diets that may require supplements, but is there an argument to be made for supplements in the absence of such conditions?

The Lewin group, based in Virginia, carries out statistical modeling and analysis for government agencies. In a study published in 2005 they estimated that dietary supplementation with omega 3 fatty acids by seniors over the age of 65, could prevent 400,000 heart disease related visits to hospitals and physicians over a five-year period and dietary supplementation with lutein and zeaxanthin could help to reduce visual loss in 100,000 adults.

Recent research has shown that supplementation with fish oil (omega 3) improves the exercise response of people with asthma.

Coenzyme Q10 is produced in the body and is important for metabolism. Levels are reduced with ageing and with certain medications, particularly cholesterol lowering drugs. There is some evidence that supplementation may have a modest effect on reducing high blood pressure. It has been suggested for heart disease, heart failure and a number of other conditions, but there is no good evidence at this time to support its use as a supplement.

We live in a heavily polluted environment that exposes us to high levels of oxidative stress. Reduction in the ozone layer exposes us to increased ultraviolet radiation. Combustion engine exhaust fumes, cigarette smoke, and industrial pollutants, all produce free radicals that pollute the atmosphere. The body therefore requires high levels of antioxidants to protect itself from free radical damage.

Agricultural practices may reduce the presence of some soil nutrients and trace minerals unless they are replaced on a regular basis, which in turn would decrease the nutritional value of the food grown. Selenium is an example of a trace mineral that is found in very low levels in some soils.

Foods are often harvested before they are ripe so that they can be transported without spoiling. As a result they do not acquire their full complement of vitamins and minerals. Nutrients may also deteriorate during transportation and storage, for instance fruits and vegetables can lose vitamin C.

Produce is often sprayed with pesticides that are harmful to health, and have the ability to accumulate in fat, hence the move towards organic produce. It is not practical in most situations to only eat locally grown organic produce year round, so we will be exposed to variable nutrient content and toxins in our food. Supplementation therefore should not necessarily be ruled out as part of, or as an addition to, a good diet.

Sweeteners

Sugar is the most commonly used sweetener, but has a high glycemic index and provides empty calories. It is present in soft drinks, and many breakfast cereals, as well as being added to tea and coffee. Many people therefore use sugar substitutes in an effort to reduce their calorie intake, either because they have diabetes or are trying to lose weight. I attended a conference on heart health recently where this topic was discussed in detail. The evidence available shows that artificial sweeteners do not reduce overall sugar intake, do not lead to weight loss and may actually lead to an increase in weight.

Saccharin was discovered in 1879, and was the first sweetener discovered. It is three hundred times as sweet as sugar, and is often mixed with aspartame. Its use is banned in Canada because of concerns that it may cause bladder cancer, but it is available in the USA.

Cyclamates were the next chemical sweeteners to be discovered and were used to mask the bitter taste of some medications. They are thirty to fifty time sweeter than sugar and often mixed with saccharin. They were banned in 1969 by the food and drug administration because of a possible connection to the development of bladder cancer and testicular atrophy, however, they are still used in many parts of the world, where they are sold under the names of Sucaryl and Sweet'N Low.

Aspartame was the next sweetener to be discovered, in 1965 by Searle. It is one hundred and eighty times sweeter than sugar, but has the disadvantage of breaking down when heated, and cannot therefore be used in cooking. There has been much controversy surrounding the safety of aspartame, with regard to the development of brain tumors, lymphoma (a type of cancer), and possibly multiple sclerosis, but currently it has been approved as safe for human consumption in over ninety countries around the world, and is sold as NutraSweet. It is interesting to note that one hundred percent of the industry funded research (74 trials) attests to the safety of aspartame, where as 92 percent of independently funded research (92 trials) identified a safety concern.

Scientists working for Tate and Lyle in London England discovered Sucralose in 1976. It is six hundred times sweeter than sugar and is sold under the brand name Splenda. Sucralose is heat stable and therefore suitable for use in baked goods. Most of the Sucralose ingested is not absorbed, being excreted in the feces. The small amount that is absorbed is largely eliminated in urine by the kidneys. Most regulatory bodies have accepted Sucralose as being safe, and it is the only artificial sweetener to be ranked as safe by the Center for Science in the Public Interest.

Stevia is a genus of numerous species of herbs and shrubs in the sunflower family, native to South and Central America. Stevia rebaudiana is widely grown for its sweet leaves, which have been used medicinally by the Guarani tribes in Paraguay and Brazil for several centuries as a treatment for heartburn and other ailments. Recent research has shown promise in its use for treating obesity, high blood pressure, osteoporosis, and as a sweetener for diabetics.

Stevia extracts are three hundred times sweeter than sugar, and have been used as sweeteners in Japan since 1971. Stevia is available in Canada as a dietary supplement. Stevia is a natural product and cannot be patented, therefore having less commercial appeal, which may be the reason that it is having difficulty being approved as a sweetener in many countries. One could ask the question as to why it is safe as a supplement and not as a sweetener?

In my opinion the sweetener of choice is sugar, and for those who wish to avoid the calories that come with sugar, Stevia would seem to be a good alternative.

Adaptogens

The term adaptogen refers to a natural herb product that is proposed to increase the body's resistance to stress, trauma, anxiety and fatigue. All adaptogens contain antioxidants, but that is not thought to be their primary mode of action.

An adaptogen has three properties.

1. An adaptogen is non-toxic.
2. An adaptogen produces a nonspecific response in the body—an increase in the power of resistance against multiple stressors including physical, chemical or biological agents.
3. An adaptogen has a normalizing influence on physiology, irrespective of the direction of change from physiological norms caused by the stressor.

It is claimed that adaptogenic herbs are distinct from other substances in their ability to balance endocrine hormones and the immune system, and that they help to maintain optimal homeostatsis by toning down overactivity, or increasing underactivity in the body's systems. There are fourteen definite and ten probable herbs known to have these properties. Common examples are red gingseng from Asia, white American ginseng, Siberian ginseng, Suma, ashwaganda, astragalus, licorice, schisandra and jiaogulan. Reishi, shiitake and maitake mushrooms are also considered to have adaptogenic properties. Many of these herbs have been used in traditional Chinese medicine for centuries, and are just recently being investigated by western medicine.

Salba

A recent study from St. Michael's Hospital in Toronto carried out by V. Vuksan et al., published in 2007, showed that the addition of two tablespoons of salba per day to the diet, significantly reduced systolic blood pressure, high-sensitivity C-reactive protein and Von Willebrand factor (all risk markers for coronary artery disease) in patients with type two diabetes, beyond conventional therapy, while maintaining good control of blood sugar and blood fats.

Salba is a truly remarkable food source. It contains gram for gram, eight times more omega 3 than salmon, four times more fiber than flax, six times more calcium than whole milk, thirteen times more antioxidants than blueberries, has no trans-fats, and very few carbohydrates.

According to ancient manuscripts dating back to 3500 B.C., salba was an important nutritional component of the Aztec diet, and was called "running food," because their messengers were said to be able to run all day on a handful of the seeds.

It can be obtained in powder or seed form, and either used in baking or sprinkled over cereal. It has very little taste and tends to take on the flavor of whatever it is eaten with. The seeds have to be ground, or they will pass through the intestine intact and their nutritional value lost.

Probiotics

A probiotic is a substance that contains live micro-organisms which when ingested in adequate amounts, confer a health benefit.

Yogurt is an example of a probiotic, but not all yogurts have been shown to have probiotic effects. The cheapest and most easily obtainable probiotic yogurt is Activia made by Danone. Other probiotic substances that have been shown to have health benefits are Align, Danactive probiotic drink, Tuzen, Bio-K+cl1285, and Rephresh proB. These substances have been shown to be beneficial in the treatment of diarrhea, irritable bowel syndrome, inflammatory bowel disease, vaginal infections and in enhancing immunity.

Dark Chocolate seems to be a good food to finish this section with. Dark chocolate by definition has more than 65% cacao. It contains antioxidants, tends to lower blood pressure by increasing nitric oxide, which relaxes the arteries, lowers LDL (the bad fat), stimulates the release of endorphins and increases the production of serotonin in the brain, both of which are mood enchancers. The recommended dose is not more 3–4 ounces per day.

> Eat a plant-based diet with lots of fruits and vegetables.
> Limit intake of red meat and animal fat. Eat lean meat and poultry. 4 oz servings.
> Eat fish twice a week.

4
Exercising

Exercise is a form of physical activity. Physical activity may be broadly defined as activity that encompasses all forms of muscle movements, that can range from sports to lifestyle activities. Exercise may be defined as physical activity, which is planned, structured movement of the body designed to enhance physical fitness. There are three types of exercise: stretching, aerobic and anaerobic.

Stretching is a form of exercise designed to maintain and enhance flexibility. Flexibility refers to the range of motion in a joint or group of joints, and depends on the elasticity of the muscles and tendons around the joints. As people age, the muscles and tendons tend to lose their elasticity, making it difficult to perform everyday tasks, as range of motion decreases. Regular stretching therefore becomes increasingly important as we get older, in order to maintain as much elasticity as possible.

Flexibility is important for activities of daily living. Maintaining flexibility helps to reduce falls and injuries, enables us to bend down to pick things up from the ground, and makes it easier to get in and out of vehicles.

Stretching should be a daily, life long activity, and is best done when the muscles are warm, after doing some gentle calisthenics or aerobic exercise. There are many stretching exercises and they can be tailored to specific forms of activity, but the following stretching regimen is suitable for general purposes.

During aerobic exercise, work is accomplished by utilizing oxygen to produce energy, whereas with anaerobic exercise, energy is produced without utilizing oxygen. These two types of exercise use different chemical processes for energy production. These differences are important, because anaerobic exercise results in production of lactic acid, and oxygen debt, and is therefore of relatively short duration, as the body has limited ability to tolerate lactic acid, and oxygen debt.

Aerobic exercise on the other hand can be of extended duration, as long as there is fuel and oxygen available to produce energy. Whilst these two forms of exercise are distinct, they often coexist, and are part of a continuum. The intensity and duration of the exercise determines which form of energy production is paramount. In a progressive exercise situation, where the intensity of the exercise steadily increases from low to high, initial energy production will be aerobic, but as the intensity increases, there comes a point at which the heart and lungs are not able to supply all of the oxygen required to meet the increasing energy demand, and anaerobic work will begin to take place. If the energy requirement continues to increase, there will come a time when all further energy production will be anaerobic, and the person will soon become exhausted and have to stop.

When we carry out a graded maximal exercise test, measuring the oxygen uptake (VO2) and the amount of air being breathed (Ve), we can demonstrate the changeover from aerobic to anaerobic metabolism by plotting the Ve against VO2 on a graph. At first VO2 and Ve have a linear relationship, increasing proportionally, but as the test continues Ve begins to increase at a more rapid rate than VO2, indicating that lactic acid production is starting to increase. The dis-

Stretching

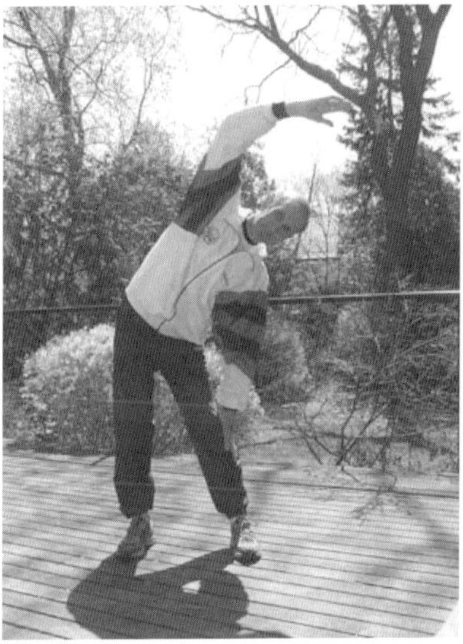

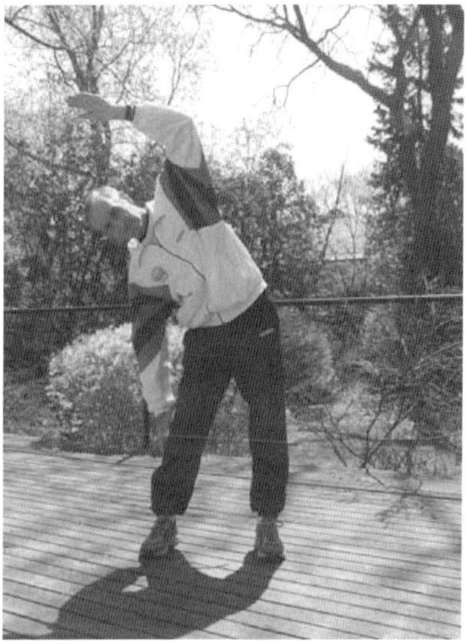

Side Bends

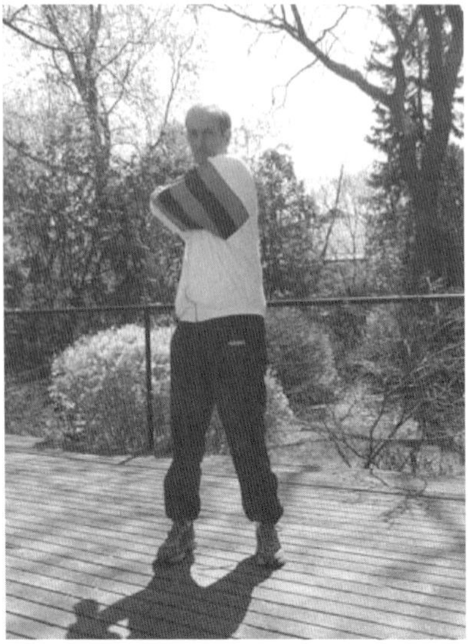

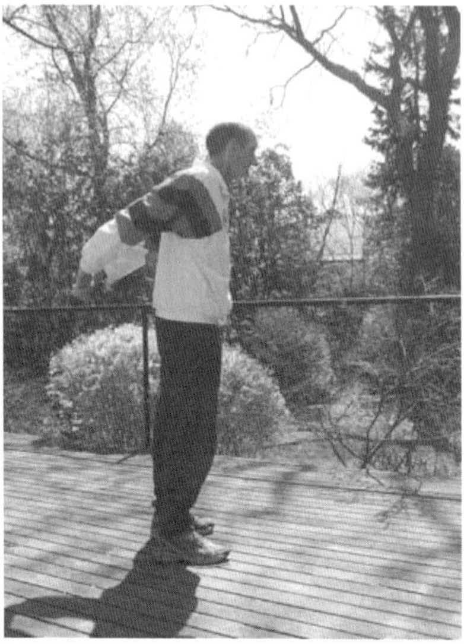

Shoulder Stretches

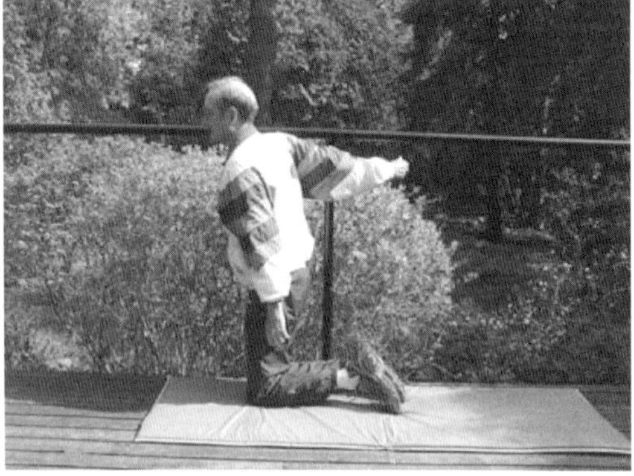

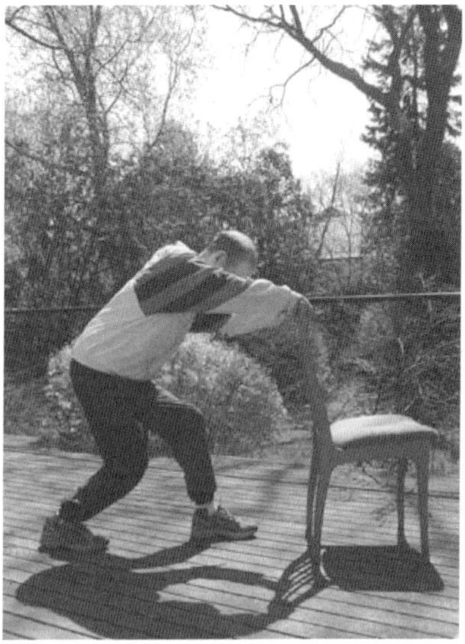

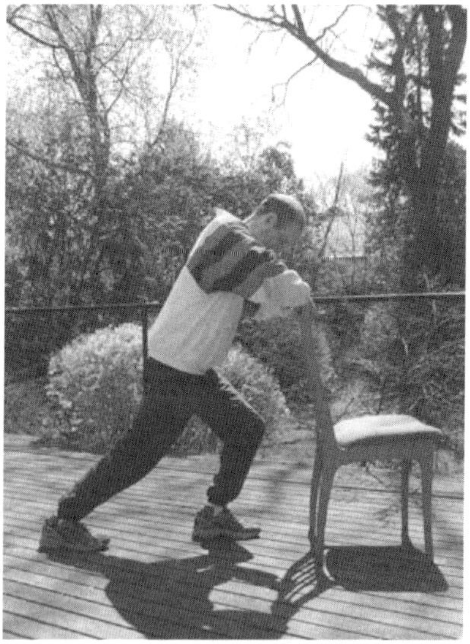

Achilles

Calf

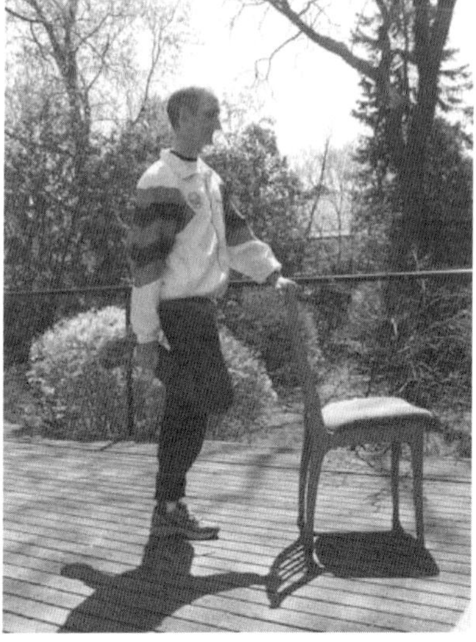

Thigh

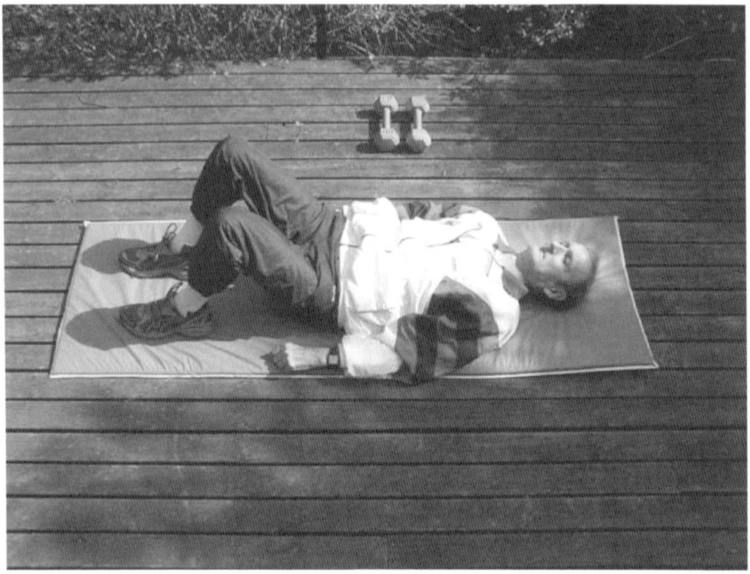

lower back

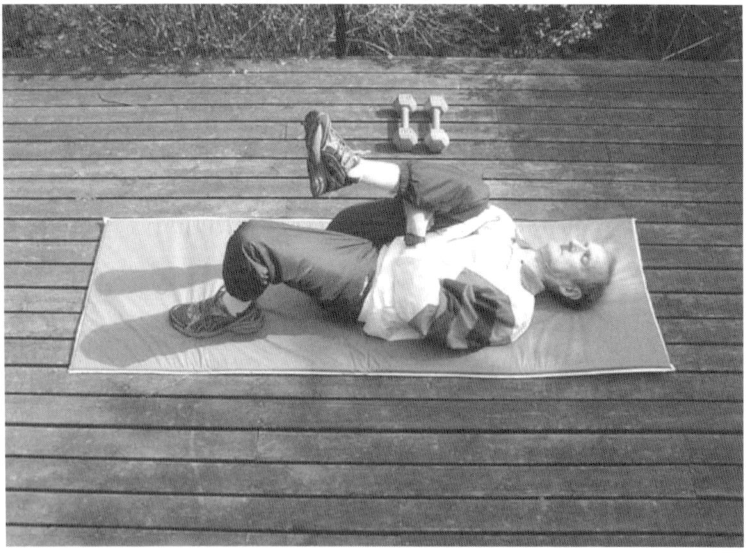

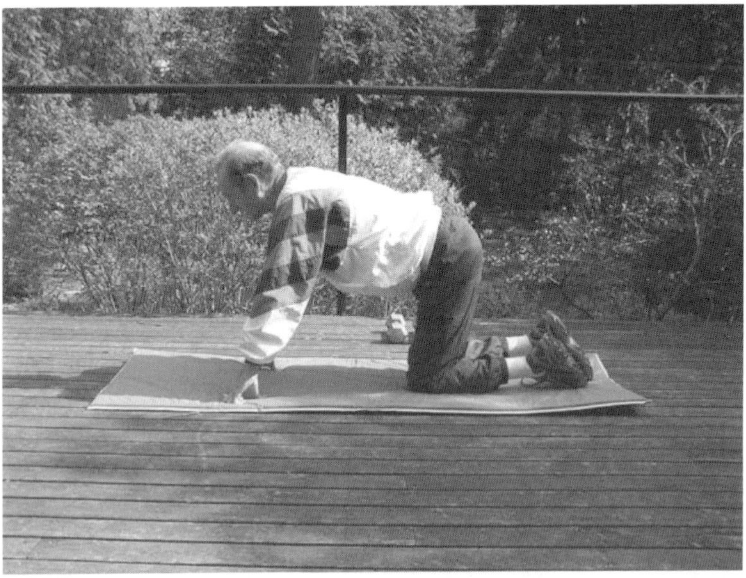

Bird Dog

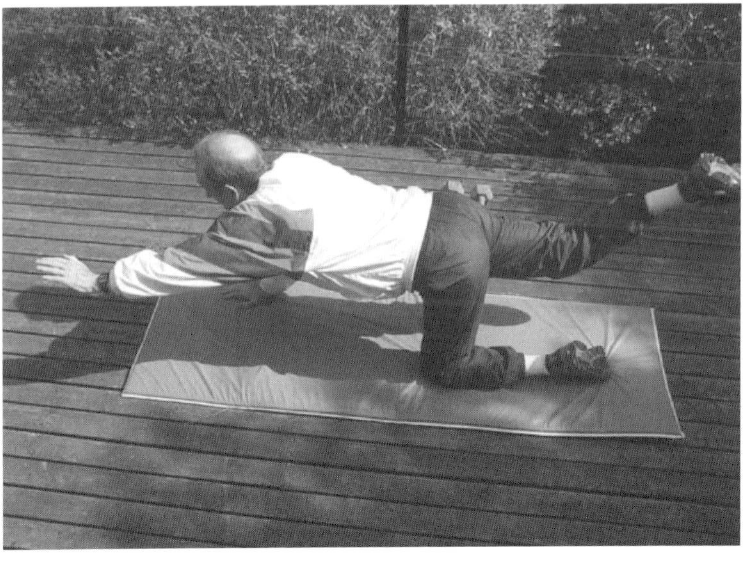

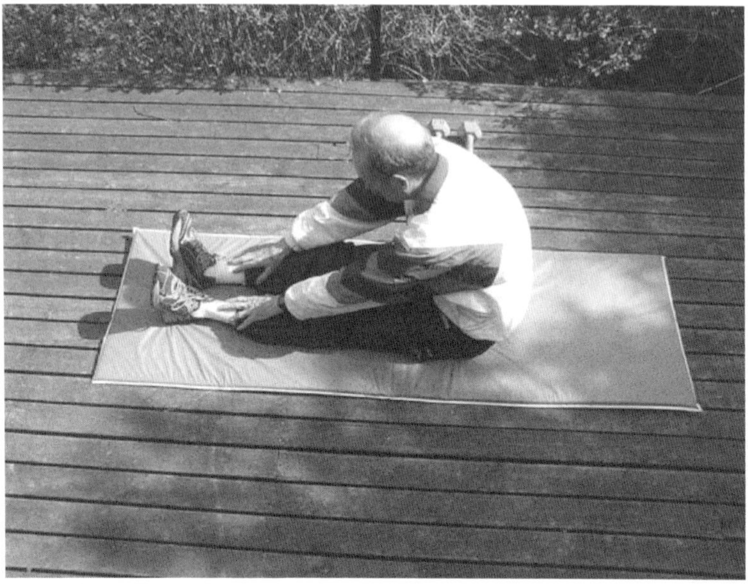

Sit and Reach

proportionate increase in Ve allows more carbon dioxide to be expelled, which helps the body to tolerate the increasing lactic acid production.

Blood has a buffering system to keep the acidity (pH) at a constant level. Carbon dioxide is produced during energy production, and is buffered by (combined with) bicarbonate to prevent the pH of the blood from changing. When lactic acid production increases during anaerobic metabolism, carbon dioxide is given off so that the bicarbonate can buffer lactic acid, and the carbon dioxide that is released is associated with an increase in Ve.

The graph shows two break points from the original linear relationship. The first breakpoint, when Ve starts to increase faster than VO2, indicates the point at which some of the increase in energy required is being produced anaerobically, and the second break point, where the Ve is increasing with little or no increase in VO2, represents the point at which all the increase in energy production is accomplished anaerobically. These break points are called thresholds, and occur at approximately 2 and 4 mmol of blood lactate. The first threshold has several names. The name that I prefer is the ventilatory threshold (VT), although many others call it the anaerobic threshold (AT). The second threshold is usually called the respiratory compensation point (RCP).

Maximal VO2 is the international measurement of fitness, and determines how much physical work an individual is capable of doing. The higher the VO2, the more work a person is capable of, and the fitter the person is said to be. The ability of a person to take up oxygen is trainable within limits, which are usually genetically determined. The amount of improvement that can be obtained is also dependant on how fit a person is to start with. A person starting with a low level of fitness will generally obtain a greater degree of improvement with training than a person starting with a high level of fitness.

VO2 is expressed in two ways, absolute and relative. Absolute VO2 is measured in liters per minute (L.min), and will be influenced by stature and muscle mass. Relative VO2 is related to body mass and is expressed as milliliters per kilogram per minute (ml.kg.min). Relative VO2 is more meaningful in describing what an individual is capable of doing. For instance a very large person with an absolute VO2 of 4 L. min may only have a relative VO2 of 20 ml.kg. min. Compared to a smaller person with an absolute VO2 of 4L.min and a relative VO2 of 40 ml.kg.min. Both have the same absolute VO2, but one is much fitter than the other.

All physical work that we do requires the uptake of oxygen, so the greater the ability to take up oxygen the easier

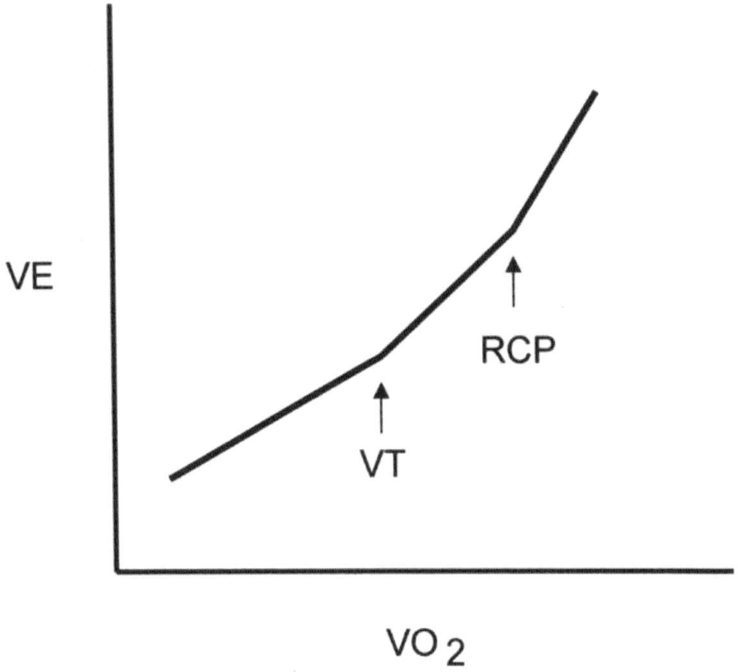

Figure 7. Graph of VO2 vs. Ve

a given amount of work will be. For example if a person's maximum VO2 is 50 ml.kg.min and the task requires an oxygen uptake of 20 ml.kg.min. That person will be working 40% of maximum capacity, but if maximum VO2 is only 25 ml.kg.min that person will be working at 80% of maximum capacity, and the work will seem much harder even though the task is the same.

In a study of 12,169 men referred for cardiac rehabilitation published in *Circulation,* we showed that VO2 max at entry to the program was the best predictor of both all cause and cardiac mortality. Follow up was 4 to 29 years with a median of 7.9 years. Men with a max VO2 of >22 ml.kg.min had a 0.45 and 0.39 risk of all cause and cardiac death over the period of observation compared to those with a max VO2 of <15 ml.kg.min. There is no reason to believe that this would not also be true for healthy individuals, as max VO2 is a reflection of genetic inheritance and life style.

Physical fitness has four components, cardiovascular fitness, muscular strength, muscular endurance and flexibility. To improve and maintain flexibility we use stretching exercises as discussed earlier. To improve and maintain cardiovascular fitness we use aerobic training, and to improve and maintain muscular strength and endurance we use resistance training.

Training cardiovascular fitness for most people will require aerobic exercise, but athletes will do a considerable amount of anaerobic training as well, as their goals are different. When considering a regular exercise-training program there are four important components that follow a simple mnemonic FITT. The F is for frequency, I is for intensity, and the Ts stand for time and type of exercise.

The recommended frequency varies from three times per week to daily, depending on the source. Many cardiac rehabilitation programs in the USA have patients exercise three times a week, whereas in Canada five times a week is more common. The American College of Sports medicine (ACSM) recommends that the general population exercise on most days of the week. I personally believe that we should exercise every day whenever possible.

Intensity is the most difficult component to accurately prescribe for the general population. VO2 max can be used to prescribe the intensity of exercise. The ACSM recommends an intensity of 50 to 80% of maximum VO2, but how does a person know what that intensity is without having an exercise test to measure their maximum VO2? Clearly an exercise test to measure maximum VO2 is ideal, but impractical and too expensive for the general population, although frequently done for patients with heart disease who are entered into rehabilitation programs, and for athletes.

Heart rate is another method frequently used to prescribe exercise intensity. The ACSM recommends 60 to 90% of maximal heart rate as being an appropriate exercise intensity, but this approach has several drawbacks.

Maximal heart rate is estimated from formulae based on age, the most common and simple being 220 minus the person's age. Unfortunately this may vary by plus or minus 15 beats, and is altered by a number of medications, most notably the beta-blockers that are frequently used to treat high blood pressure.

Not everyone is able to take their pulse accurately, and the heart rate slows very quickly when exercise stops, so this method though widely used, has problems. If you choose to use this method then you should count the number of beats in ten seconds and multiply by six, so as to minimize the effect of the rapid slowing of the heart rate. Another method is to use the Borg Rating of Perceived Exertion Scale. (RPE)

This scale as you can see starts at 6 and goes to 20 with a verbal description beside some of the numbers. Borg, in

Sweden, using young healthy students, originally developed this scale, and the numbers multiplied by ten corresponded to the heart rate. As people age their maximal heart rate decreases, so the numbers no longer reflect the actual heart rate, but continue to reflect the relative effort, so it remains useful. Exercising at a perceived exertion of about 13 (somewhat hard) is an appropriate intensity for most people, as long as their perception is normal. Unfortunately it is my experience that some people either have a disorder of perception or do not tell the truth. I have tested people who reach maximum VO2 and will tell me that their RPE is only 12 when it is quite obvious that they cannot do any more work, and others who will happily continue to exercise at an RPE of 20 for several minutes.

Some years ago Professor Bob Goode at the University of Toronto proposed the talk test, as a result of a conversation with a mountain climber who told him that it was common for climbers to climb only as fast as they could carry on a conversation. More recently my son Robert, while doing his masters degree with Dr. Goode, showed that the level of exertion at which you can first hear your breathing corresponds to the beginning of anaerobic work. This intensity corresponds to the VT, which is usually associated with an RPE of 12 or 13 on the Borg scale, and has been named the breath sound check. The talk test is associated with slightly higher exercise intensity, but is still within the safe yet effective training intensity range. The breath sound check and the talk test have been validated by other researchers, and are in my opinion, the simplest reliable guide to exercise intensity available to the general population.

The breath sound check has the advantage of correlating very closely with VT, which varies from person to person from 40 to 80% of VO2 max. It therefore allows for an accurate prescription of exercise intensity for any individual.

Borg Scale

6

7 Extremely Light

8

9 Very Light

10

11 Light

12

13 Somewhat Hard

14

15 Hard

16

17 Very Hard

18

19 Extremely Hard

20 Maximal Exertion

The Borg scale

In general the higher the intensity of exercise, the shorter is the duration required to get a training effect, and the lower the intensity, the greater the duration of exercise that is required.

Time or duration of exercise has been the subject of much research, and recommendations will vary according to the intensity of exercise, and the goals of the exerciser. ACSM recommends that the average adult should get between 150 and 250 minutes of moderate intensity exercise per week. What qualifies as moderate intensity depends on age and fitness level, and will usually be between 3 and 10 METS. MET is shorthand for metabolic equivalent, and is supposed to be the amount of oxygen that a person takes up at complete rest, usually quoted as being 3.5 ml.kg.min. This is a generally accepted number, but it should be noted that it does vary from person to person. This definition of moderate intensity exercise spans a range of VO2 between 10.5 and 35 ml.kg.min. Walking at 18 minutes per mile (3.33 mph) requires a VO2 of about 15 ml.kg.min, which is quite a slow pace, unless you are unfit, whereas a VO2 of 35 ml.kg.min would allow for jogging.

150 to 250 minutes per week translates into approximately 20 to 35 minutes per day of exercise. This is probably a realistic goal for sedentary people who need to get started on doing something, but in my opinion is not sufficient for optimal health benefits. ACSM recognizes that in order to lose weight, a greater duration of exercise is necessary, and recommends 225 to 300 minutes per week. This translates into approximately 32 to 43 minutes per day. This recommendation is supported by my own research with overweight cardiac patients, who lost an average of 4.5 kg, with a walking program averaging 43 minutes a day, 7 days a week. The weight loss was maintained over one year.

I believe the goal for most people should be 30 to 60

minutes of exercise, preferably daily, with a minimum of 5 days per week.

Type of exercise should allow for individual preferences, but in general would include activities that use large muscle groups, can be maintained continuously, and are rhythmical and aerobic in nature. Examples would include activities such as walking, hiking, jogging, skipping, rowing, stair climbing, swimming, skating, racquet sports and golf (walking).

Muscular strength is the maximal amount of force that muscle can exert with a single maximal effort. Muscular strength is important for activities of everyday living, and is necessary for independent living. Muscular strength can be improved with strength training, even in the very old, and is associated with the ability to get in and out of a chair, ability to climb stairs and with walking pace. Muscular strength also maintains posture and protects joints from injury.

Muscular endurance is the ability of a muscle to perform repetitive contractions over time, and is also important for the performance of everyday activities without undue fatigue and discomfort.

Muscular strength and muscular endurance training requires a form of exercise training referred to as resistance training. With this type of training a person repetitively lifts weights either using machines or free weights. Each lifting of the weight is called a repetition (rep for short). After doing a set number of continuous reps, it is usual to take a short rest before repeating the process. Each completed number of continuous reps is called a set.

The number of reps in a set is determined by the goal. If the goal is strength, the reps would be few and the sets would be high, using a heavy weight. If the goal is endurance, reps would be high and the sets would be low, using a lesser weight. For most people the goal would be both strength and endurance. Typically this would call for 2 or 3 sets of 10 to 15 reps with moderate weight, 2 to 3 days week.

A common method for determining how much weight should be lifted is to find the maximum weight that can be lifted with proper form, once. This is called a 1-rep max (1RM). Once this has been established, a weight that is 60% of the 1RM is selected as the weight to be lifted, and the number of reps would begin at 10 and increase to 15 over time, as strength and endurance increase, beginning with one set, and increasing to 2 or 3 sets over time. When 15 reps can be accomplished comfortably, the weight can be increased and the reps reduced to 10, gradually increasing to 15.

Resistance training depends on the principle of overloading and actually disrupts muscle fibers, which then repair themselves and in the process become stronger. For this reason recovery time for repair is vital, and resistance training should always allow for a day of rest between sessions, to give the muscle fibers a chance to be repaired. It is also the reason that some muscle soreness is normally felt after beginning a resistance-training program. This soreness usually disappears after a couple of days.

Resistance training becomes more important as we age, because while most of us use our legs extensively, we do not get much upper body activity in our normal day-to-day lives, and quickly start to have problems with opening jars and other useful but mundane activities.

A good fitness program will have a number of components that include a warm up, both aerobic and resistance training, as well as stretching. These components do not necessarily have to be done all in one session.

Exercise for health does not have to be taken as a formal training program, but can be something as simple as going for a walk every day.

Resistance training, however, does require more formality, as it requires some equipment in order to do it. Joining a gym is a good solution for many, but dumbbells (free weights) at home can do the job for those people who are sufficiently motivated. In some respects free weights have an advantage over machines, in that they require better balance, and are closer to what we are required to do during our daily living, plus machines are expensive and free weights can be purchased at very reasonable cost.

Exercise beneficially affects all of the organs and systems within the body. ACSM has recently stated that "exercise is medicine," but unlike other medicines it has no deleterious side effects when done properly.

Cardiovascular System

There are two different nerves controlling the rate at which the heart beats, parasympathetic (vagal) nerves which slow and sympathetic nerves which speed up the heartbeat. Regular exercise causes the vagal nerves to become more active and the sympathetic nerves to become less active, thereby slowing the heartbeat. These nerves also influence the tone and reactions of the blood vessels, and as a result blood pressure is reduced after acute and regular exercise.

The work that the heart has to do is to a great degree determined by how often it has to contract (heart rate, HR), and how much pressure it has to generate in order to expel blood into the arteries (blood pressure, BP). HR multiplied by BP is called the double product and is a measure of the work that the heart is doing at any given time. Since regular exercise leads to a lower HR and BP both at rest and any given level of exercise, it stands to reason that the heart is

Simple resistance training exercises

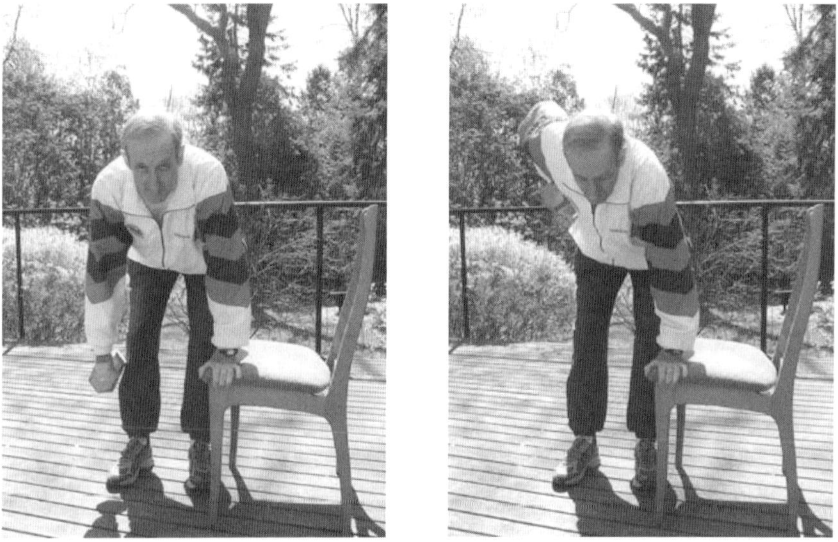

Dumbell Row

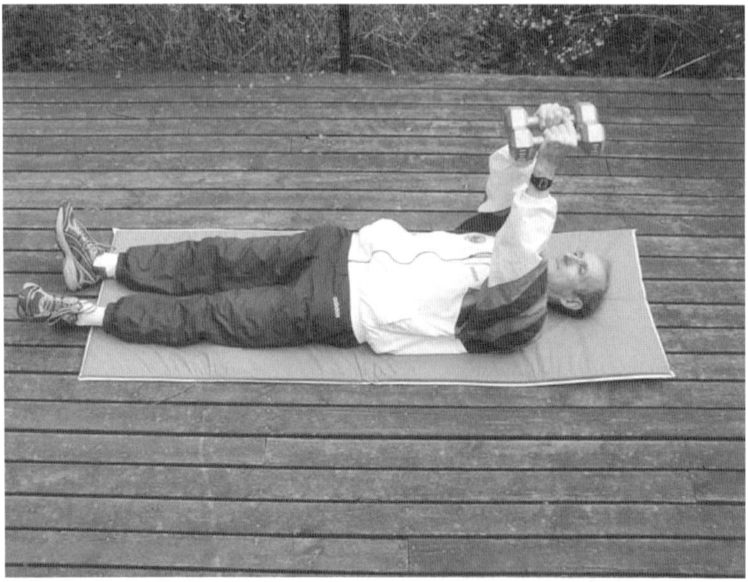

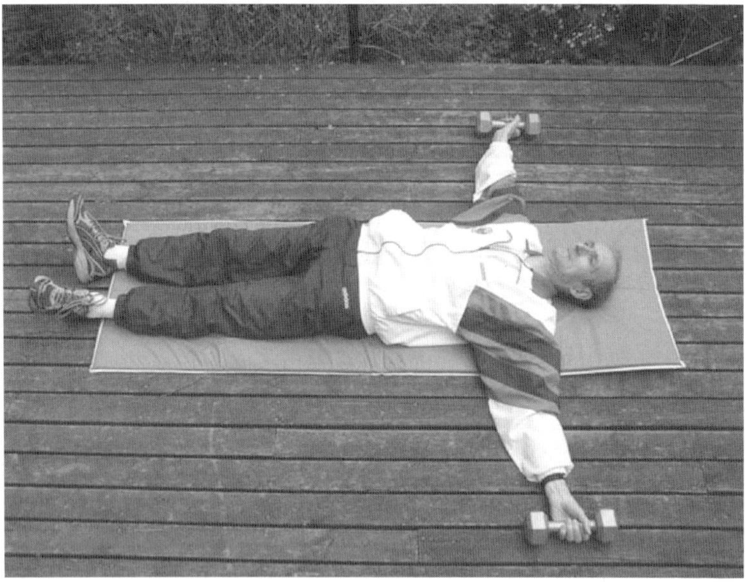

Flies

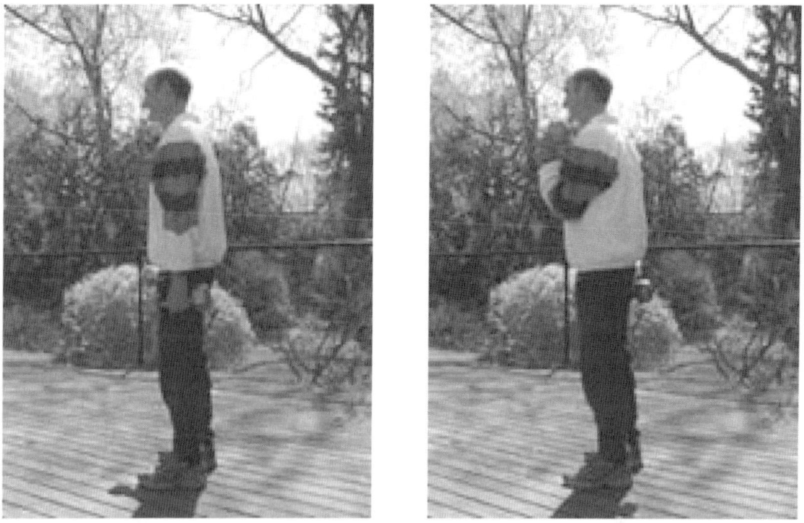

Bicep Curl

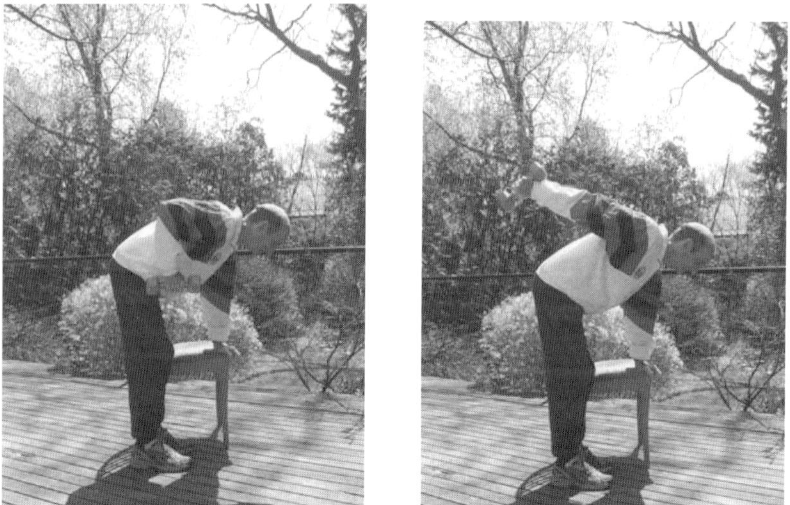

Triceps Extension

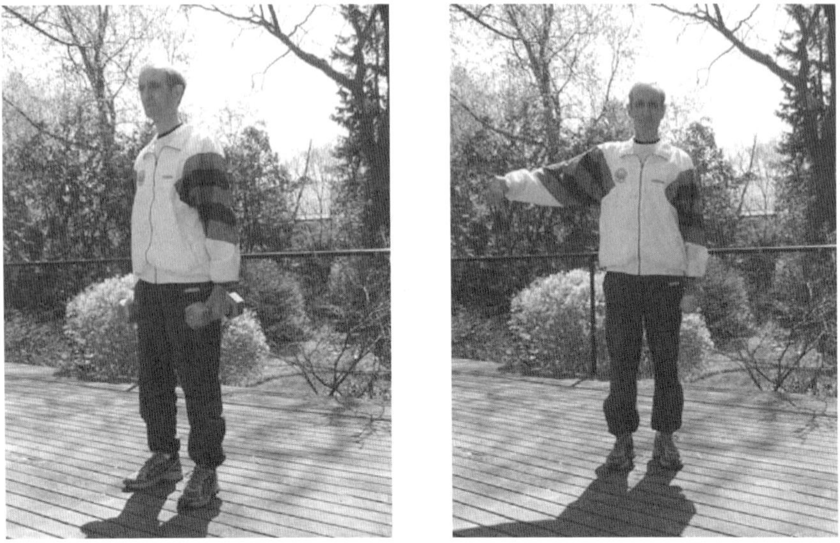

Lateral Raises

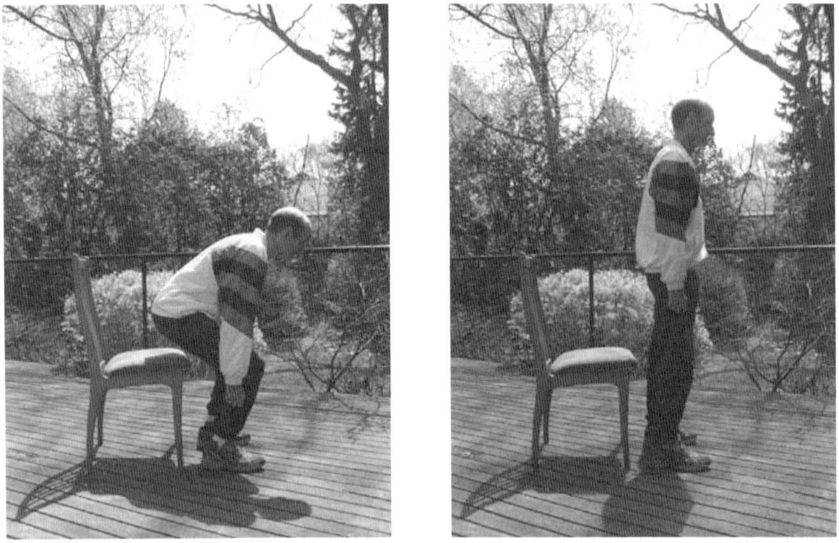

Squats

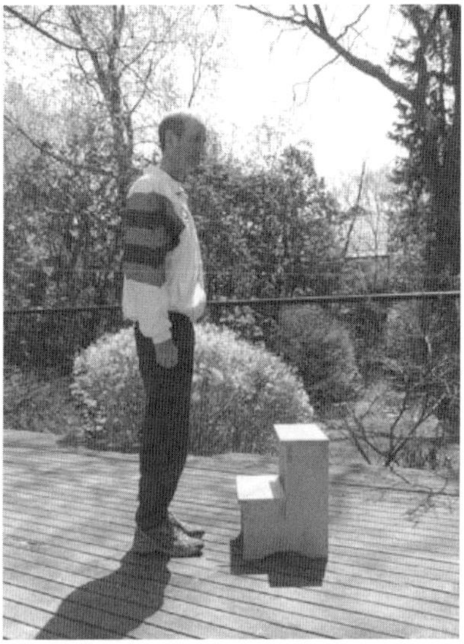

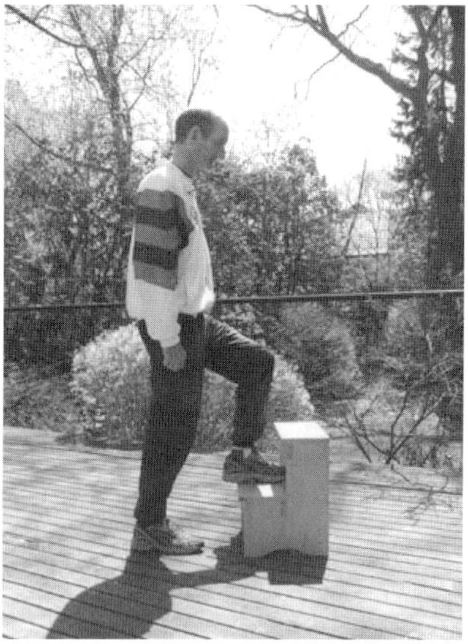

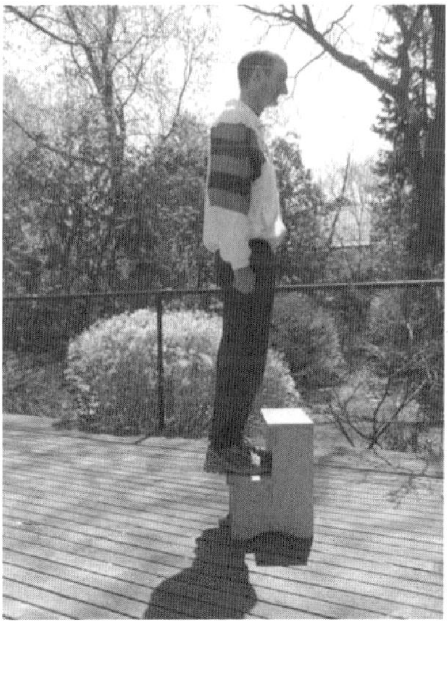

Stepping

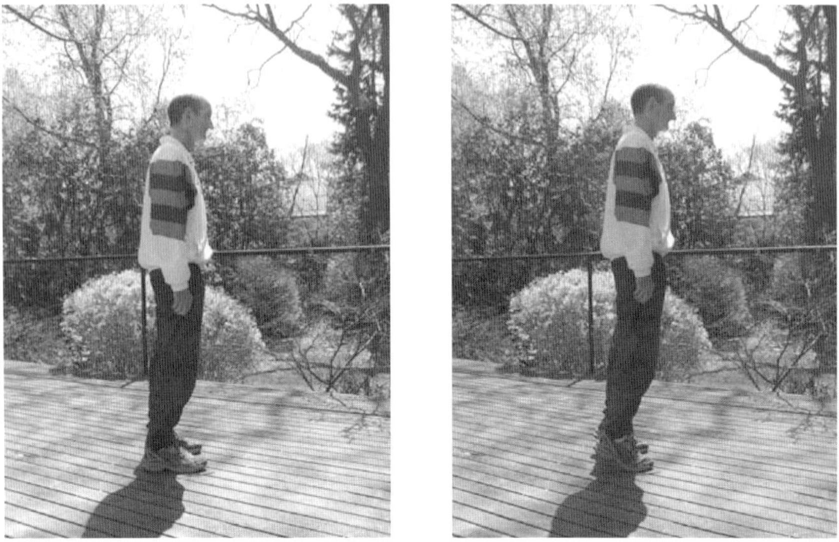

Toe Raises

doing less work at rest and at any given level of sub-maximal work.

The heart muscle is supplied with oxygen from blood flowing through the coronary arteries. Most of this blood enters the heart muscle during the time that it is relaxed (diastole), as opposed to when the muscle is contracting (systole). The slower the heart rate, the longer diastole, and the greater the supply of blood and oxygen to the heart muscle.

The heart is a pump made of muscle. It is divided into four chambers, two upper chambers called atria and two lower chambers called ventricles. The atria collect blood returning from the body and pass it into the ventricles. The right ventricle pumps blood through the lungs where it absorbs oxygen and gives off carbon dioxide. The left ventricle pumps the oxygenated blood around the body to supply cells with oxygen and nutrients.

Vigorous exercise training over time has been shown to increase the left ventricular volume by as much as 30% and to increase the thickness of the ventricular wall. These changes result in increased filling of the heart, and a more forceful contraction to expel the blood. The amount of blood expelled with each contraction is called the stoke volume (SV), and is increased after vigorous training. SV multiplied by HR is the volume of blood pumped by the heart in a given time, and is called the cardiac output (CO). An increase in SV allows the heart to maintain the same CO at a slower HR.

The enlargement of the heart produced by vigorous exercise training is associated with specific changes on the ECG, and is called athlete's heart. Historically these changes were considered to be dangerous, and led by physicians to advise against prolonged strenuous exertion.

Clarence DeMar won seven Boston Marathons and a bronze medal in the Paris Olympic games, but was advised

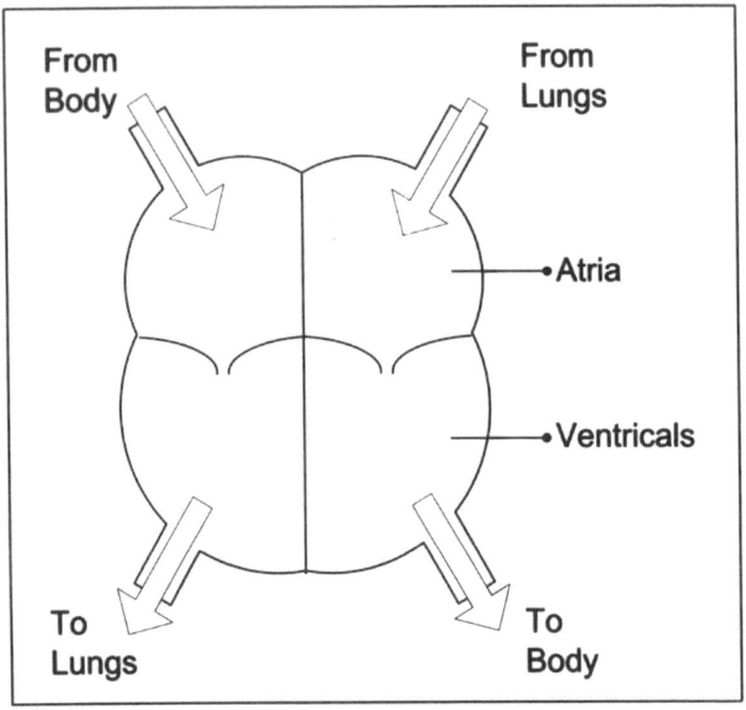

Cartoon of the heart

more than once that he should stop running as it was injurious to his health. We now know that the changes are benign and indeed may be beneficial, in that a trained heart is more resistant to dangerous abnormal rhythm disturbances.

Regular exercise over time causes new capillaries (tiny blood vessels) to grow into the muscles, which allows for an increase in the amount of blood flowing into the muscle. Since oxygen is carried on hemoglobin in the red cells by the blood, more oxygen is able to get into the muscles, which enable the muscles to do more work.

Research has shown that people who exercise regularly have more flexible blood vessels than sedentary people, and are therefore less likely to have high blood pressure. Endurance exercise also improves the ability of blood vessels to dilate. This is due to increased nitric oxide production by the cells that line the inside of the blood vessels. These cells are called endothelial cells and their behavior is termed endothelial function. The development of endothelial dysfunction is the first step towards a condition known as atherosclerosis that can lead to blockage of blood vessels, causing heart attacks, and other problems.

Regular physical activity is protective against coronary artery disease. Professor Jeremy Morris in London published the first evidence for this in 1953. Professor Morris studied people working on the London double-decker buses, which at that time had both a driver and a conductor. The conductor's job was to collect the fares from the passengers, which required climbing up and down the stairs 24 times per hour (active), while the driver sat in front (sedentary) driving through the traffic. This study found that the bus drivers were three times more likely to have heart disease than the bus conductors, and had twice as many heart attacks. The bus drivers were bigger and heavier than the conductors, so the question was raised as to whether bigger heavier people chose to drive, and lighter fitter people chose to be conductors (self-selection).

A later study by Ralph Paffenbarger looked at longshoremen working on the San Francisco docks, where at that time they physically unloaded the ships. This study found that dockworkers had less heart disease and heart attacks than office workers, and that when dockworkers were promoted to office work, their risk of heart disease and heart attack increased to match that of office workers. This demonstrated that it is what you do at the time that protects you, and that protection cannot be earned and stored. The study also showed that self-selection was not responsible for the findings.

There have been many other studies done around the world looking at the effects of physical activity, and all of them show that regular physical activity is protective against heart disease.

C reactive protein is a chemical marker of inflammation in the body, and is reduced in people who are physically active. Since coronary artery disease is known to be an inflammatory disease, reduction of C reactive protein may be part of the protective effect of exercise.

Musculoskeletal System

Muscles contain small round bodies called mitochondria that are responsible for the generation of energy. They are like little furnaces, which transform glucose and oxygen into energy. The number and size of mitochondria are increased in the muscles that are involved in performing exercise, allowing the muscle to process more glucose and oxygen.

There is a glucose receptor on muscle, called glut4,

which enables the muscle to take up glucose from blood. Exercising a muscle increases the number of glut4 receptors on the muscle cells, which in turn allows the muscle to take more glucose from blood. Muscles are comprised of two distinct types of fibers, known as slow twitch and fast twitch. Fast twitch fibers are subdivided into three groups. Slow fibers are affected by and used in endurance exercise and fast fibers are responsible for strength and short bursts of high power activity. Marathon runners have predominantly slow fibers that are good for aerobic metabolism, and sprinters have predominantly fast fibers, that are good for anaerobic metabolism. The different fiber types respond to different training stimuli, and can be trained independently. Regular exercise increases the size and strength of muscle fibers.

Bones are an important part of the musculoskeletal system, and they too respond to regular exercise. Bones are in a constant state of remodeling and respond to stresses placed upon them. A good example is seen in professional tennis players, where the bones in the dominant forearm are larger and stronger than in the non-dominant arm, having responded to the repetitive stress placed upon them by striking the ball. Older people who are physically active are less likely to suffer from osteoporosis than their sedentary counterparts. All weight bearing exercise stresses bone, and helps to maintain its structural integrity, but resistance training exercise is the most efficacious.

Swimming on the other hand, since it is not weight bearing, is not an effective form of exercise for maintaining bone strength.

There are two components to bone strength, bone mineral density and the actual architectural structure of the bone. Bone mineral density is easily measured, but bone architecture is more difficult to assess.

Stretching exercises are important to help maintain range of motion at joints.

Respiratory System

There is no good evidence that exercise training makes much difference to lung function. In fact exercising in polluted or very cold air may actually damage the lungs, causing increased inflammation and scarring. There also seems to be a very high incidence of asthma in competitive athletes, perhaps related to increased exposure to the irritants mentioned above.

Active children and adults have superior lung function compared to their less active counterparts, but their activity levels may not cause this, rather their activity levels may be reflecting the fact that they started with better lung function. Competitive swimmers have larger lung capacities than others, but again this could be due to self-selection. There is evidence to indicate that regular exercise may slow the age-related deterioration in lung function.

Specific exercise training can improve the force and endurance of the diaphragm and intercostals muscles, and is used in the treatment of people with lung disease. The blood vessels in the lung likely respond to regular exercise in the same way as other blood vessels, but they are difficult to study, so we do not really know.

Central Nervous System

There has been a lot of very exciting work done recently on how exercise affects the central nervous system. For many years it was believed that we were born with a certain number of brain cells, which slowly died off over a lifetime, and could not be replaced. It has now been shown both in animals and humans, that exercise stimulates the production of new brain cells (neurons), in areas of the brain that are important for learning and memory. Not only are new neurons developed, but also existing neurons produce new connections to other neurons. The chemical responsible for this development is called brain derived neurotrophic factor (BDNF), and its production appears to be stimulated by exercise. Fortunately there is a limit to this process; otherwise marathon runners would end up with very large heads.

In his book *Spark*, Dr. John Ratey describes how vigorous exercise has improved academic performance within some school districts in the USA, and how students are better able to concentrate and learn immediately following vigorous exercise, compared to students who have more conventional physical education classes. It seems that exercise arouses the brain and prepares it to function more effectively.

Interaction between neurons takes place at junctions called synapses, where messages are transmitted across the gap between synapses, by chemicals (neurotransmitters).

There are a number of chemicals that are neurotransmitters. They include glutamate, gammaminobutyric (GABA), norepinephrine, serotonin and dopamine. Glutamate stimulates and GABA dampens signaling activity.

Balance between neurotransmitters is important for health. Serotonin levels have a big effect on mood, and disturbed levels can be associated with depressed mood, while dopamine is important for movement. Dopamine deficiency in a particular area of the brain is the cause of Parkinson's disease.

Interestingly we have known for some time that regular exercise is very beneficial in the treatment of clinical depression, and now we know that serotonin levels are affected by exercise. Exercise is also being used in the treatment of Parkinson's disease and Attention Deficit Disorder, both of which are affected by dopamine.

Exercise appears to have the ability to improve the balance between neurotransmitters. Stress causes damage to nerve cells, in the same way as the stress of exercise damages muscle cells. Repair of the damage leads to stronger brain cells that are more resistant to future stress.

Regular exercise is a good way to relieve stress, and reduce the reaction to future stress. I had a patient who was suffering from anxiety and depression severe enough to have warranted electroconvulsive therapy, and who was taking numerous medications without relief when I first saw her. She would get panic attacks and believe that she was going to have a heart attack. Over time, and with the prescription of gradually increasing daily exercise, she was able to stop all but one medication, which she took in reduced dosage, with a marked reduction in the frequency and severity of her panic attacks and depression. She actually ended up jogging several miles per day on a regular basis.

Regular exercise has been shown to maintain improved blood flow to the brain as we age, and as a result active older people demonstrate better cognition and less Alzheimer's disease than sedentary people.

Endocrine System

We all have a fright, fight or flight reflex that no doubt developed to help secure our survival. This reflex kicks in when we experience what appears to be a dangerous situation. Imagine walking down a dark street at night and suddenly being confronted by an individual who appears to be about to mug you. Several things happen to your body. You

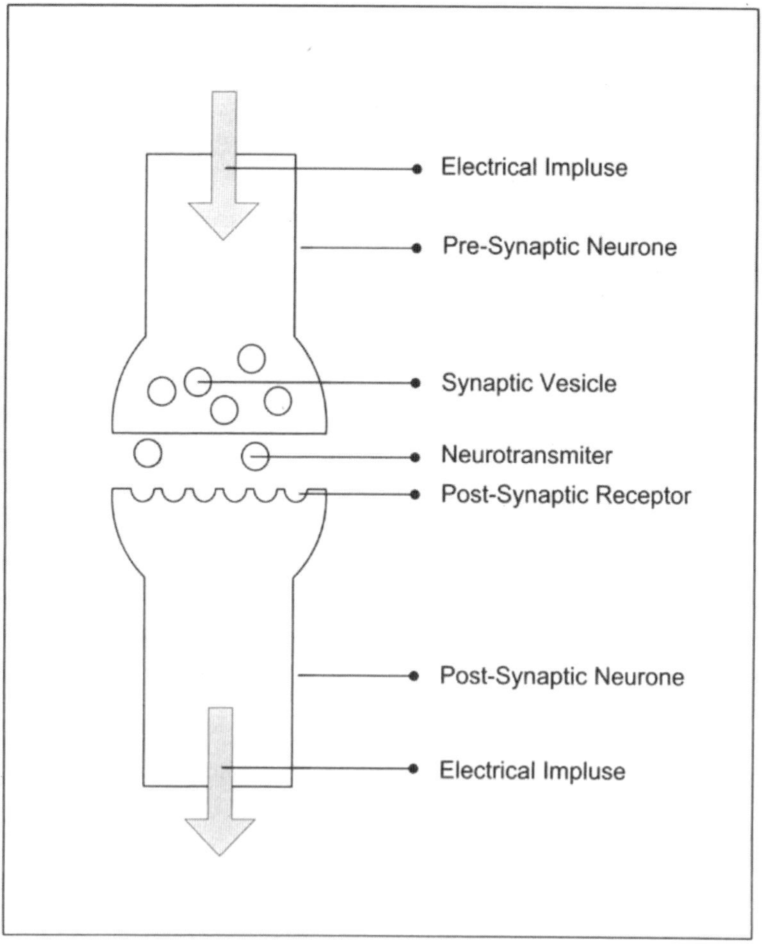

Diagram of neurons with synapses

feel your heart begin to race, you break out in a cold sweat, the hair stands up on the back of your neck, your brain becomes focused and alert, and you have a sinking feeling in the pit of your stomach. These are the things that you are consciously aware of, but a whole host of other things are happening that you do not feel. Adrenalin is released into the blood, your BP increases, blood is directed away from the skin and into your muscles, cortisol level increases, glucose is released into the blood stream and the blood becomes stickier. The increased HR, BP, blood flow to muscles, and glucose in the blood are what is needed for immediate physical exertion. Reduced blood flow to skin and stickier blood are useful in the case of injury, so that blood loss will be minimized from any wound that may be sustained. All of these changes are getting you ready for action and its consequences, whether it is to fight or to run. In this situation the physical exertion that ensues will utilize the changes, and when the episode is over all the changes will have reverted to normal. If on the other hand you are in a stressful situation that continues without the opportunity for physical release, as maybe the situation at work, all of the changes persist, and are very detrimental to health, eventually leading to diabetes, high blood pressure and or heart disease.

Regular physical activity reduces the HPA axis response to psychological stress by reducing glucocorticoid sensitivity and cortisol response.

Human growth hormone release generally follows a circadian rhythm, and is released in several discrete pulses during the cycle, the largest pulse being about one hour following the onset of sleep. Exercise above VT is a major stimulus to the release of growth hormone.

Diet also plays a part, with carbohydrate tending to reduce and protein tending to increase secretion of growth hormone in response to exercise.

There is contradictory evidence concerning the effect of exercise on the secretion of insulin like growth factor (IGF-1). A recent study done on breast cancer survivors found a reduction of IGF-1 following moderate intensity aerobic exercise training. Since breast cancer is associated with higher insulin and IGF-1 levels this is potentially beneficial. Another recent study looked at the effect of combined strength and aerobic training in elderly women, mean age sixty-six years, and found an increase in IGF-1 after training. The major difference between the two studies was strength training in the elderly women, but not in the breast cancer survivors. Now we need to know whether strength training might adversely affect breast cancer survivors.

A recent study from Berkeley, California, found that benign prostatic hypertrophy (BPH) is inversely related to exercise intensity and duration. The researchers studied 28,612 men diagnosed with BPH and concluded "greater distances run per week may reduce BPH risk independent of BMI, 10-km performance and diet."

There is equivocal evidence that regular exercise may reduce the risk of prostate cancer, and good evidence that regular exercise is beneficial for men who have prostate cancer, reducing the likelihood that they will die from it.

A study from Shiraz University in Iran published in the *Journal of Gynecology and Endocrinology* in November 2008, found that a physical fitness program for female students, consisting of aerobic and strength training, significantly reduced premenstrual symptoms and menstrual cramps.

Immune System

The intensity and duration of exercise determines the effect on the immune system. Moderately intense physical activity is associated with positive changes in immune function, which over time translates to fewer upper respiratory tract infections (URTI). People who exercise regularly report fewer colds than their sedentary peers. Surveys of runners and master athletes indicate that between 60 to 90% believe that they experience fewer colds than their sedentary peers. Data from several randomized studies support the reduction of sick days in subjects who are habitually physically active.

A recent one-year study by Matthews demonstrated a 23% reduction in URTI in those engaging in regular versus irregular moderate-to-vigorous physical activity. Very vigorous and prolonged physical activity on the other hand has been associated with an increase in URTI, especially after a competition. Immunity seems to be suppressed for a period of 3 to 72 hours following very strenuous and prolonged activity.

If you have an URTI, exercise is not contra indicated, but if you have a fever, or muscle aches and pains from an infection then you should not exercise until you have been free of symptoms for at least 48 hours.

Over the years I have found regular endurance exercise in the form of walking, jogging and running to be very beneficial in handling stress. Often a problem would seem to be much less significant after a good run, my mood improved, and the problem more easily solved. There is evidence in the literature to suggest that mental function may be impaired during high intensity exercise, but I have developed many ideas for education and research while running.

Try to get at least one hour of physical activity every day.
Stretch every day, preferably after exercise.
Do resistance training three times per week.
Build physical activity into everyday living.

5
Obesity

Obesity and overweight have become such an important and prevalent problem as to warrant their own chapter.

Obesity may be defined in terms of body mass index (BMI), BMI is derived from body mass in kilograms divided by height in meters squared. BMI between 25 and 30 is overweight and BMI greater than 30 is obese. What is really important is the relationship of body fat mass to lean body mass. BMI may be misleading at times in terms of distinguishing body composition, but it is one of the simplest measures we have. The gold standard for determining the proportion of fat mass to lean mass is underwater weighing (displacement of water), which is both too time consuming and expensive for general use. There are several other methods such as body plethysmography (displacement of air), DXA (dual X-ray Absorpitometry), BIA (biomepedance analysis), and skin fold measurement, all of which require time and expensive equipment, compared to measuring height and weight.

The distribution of body fat has a significant impact on the risk for diabetes and heart disease. The simple measurement of waist circumference is favored over all other measurements by some experts, because fat around the middle is a dangerous thing to have in terms of risk to your health.

For men, a waist circumference of 40 inches or greater,

and for women a waist circumference of 35 inches or greater, is associated with an approximately 80% chance of having metabolic syndrome.

A recent study from Great Britain published in *The Lancet* found that severe obesity—a BMI of 40 to 50 (2% of the population) reduced life expectancy by about 10 years, and moderate obesity—a BMI of 30 to 39 (25% of the population) reduced life expectancy by about 3 years.

At the present time it is estimated that 34% of Americans are obese, and the rapid increase of obesity in children is very worrisome. The incidence of obesity in children age 2 to 5 increased from approximately 5% in 1980 to 14% in 2004, children age 6 to 11 from 6% to 19%, and children age 12 to 19 from 5% to 17% over the same period. It was predicted that one in three children born in 2005 would be diabetic by the time they reach adulthood. This may be the first generation to die before their parents. Obesity in children is defined as having a BMI over the 95th percentile. The figures for Great Britain are similar, and this appears to be a worldwide problem, with huge increases in India and China.

Type two diabetes used to be a disease seen in adults, but has become increasingly common in children, and is largely related to obesity, which in turn seems to be associated with lack of exercise and ready access to poor quality high calorie foods. If current trends continue, obesity-related illnesses will overwhelm the health care systems of many nations.

The Ontario Medical Association has recently called for caloric menu labeling in chain restaurants and schools in an attempt to raise awareness of calorie intake. This has been done in some jurisdictions in the USA with reported positive health effects. Many people seriously underestimate the calorie content of fast foods, and putting the calorie content on the menu helps people to make better choices.

The incidence of obesity is inversely related to the number of years of schooling, and to economic status.

The costs of obesity-related healthcare and lost working days is 45 billion dollars per year in the USA.

Homo sapiens evolved as hunter-gatherers, having to expend a great deal of energy in order to obtain their food. The diet would have included fruits, nuts, vegetable matter and lean meat or fish. Since then there have been three important revolutions. The first occurred about ten thousand years ago when Homo sapiens discovered agriculture. This discovery allowed people to live together in larger groups, move about less, and enabled some people to live off the labor of others. I suspect that prior to the advent of agriculture there was little if any obesity. Coincident with the advent of agriculture and the formation of larger stationary settlements, some people would come to own the fields and employ others to do the physical work necessary to produce crops. Some of the owners became sedentary, and started to gain weight. At that time being overweight would have been a status symbol, indicating that the person was wealthy and important. It would also have been an unrealized health risk.

The second important event was the industrial revolution, occurring a little more than one hundred years ago, which saw the invention of machines capable of replacing manual work. Tractors replaced hand plows, trains and cars replaced horses and carriages, cranes replaced manual lifting and carrying, so that nowadays it is difficult to find jobs that involve manual labor. Paffenbarger would not have been able to do his study on the San Francisco dockworkers today because the cargo is in containers lifted by cranes.

The third revolution is the advent of the computer age.

It is now possible to shop on line, requiring only the use of the mouse and keypad, further reducing physical activity. I was at the annual meeting of ACSM several years ago where a study was done on the attendee's use of the stairs versus the escalators. Initially most of the attendees used the escalators, in spite of the fact that they were all interested in exercise, sports and health. After attendees became aware of the study, more began to use the stairs. This does illustrate how exercise is engineered out of our lives, and that we become sedentary unless we make a conscious effort to remain active. Our ancient genes are in conflict with our modern lifestyle.

In order for weight to remain constant, energy in must equal energy out; one cannot manufacture something out of nothing. Put another way, food taken in must be balanced by energy output. If energy in exceeds energy out, weight will increase, and if energy out exceeds energy in, weight will decrease.

This principle goes a long way toward explaining why there has been such a large increase in the incidence of obesity, because while calorie intake has decreased over the past one hundred years, energy output has decreased even more, leaving us with a surplus of calories that have to be stored. All calories in excess of those needed for energy production, end up being stored as fat. If the excess calories are taken in as fat they can go directly into the fat storage cells, but if they are taken in as carbohydrate or protein, they have first to be converted to fat, and that process requires energy, so that not all of the excess calories will end up in storage. This means that excess calories in the form of fat are the worst kind. Also remember that one gram of fat is worth nine calories whereas one gram of carbohydrate or protein is worth only four calories.

Most of the calories burned for energy production are

burned at rest, since that is the state in which we spend the majority of our time. As a result, small changes in BMR have the potential to create large changes in calorie utilization. If we are getting adequate sleep, one third of the day is spent at complete rest, and if we follow the ACSM recommendation of 30 to 60 minutes of exercise daily, that accounts for 2.2 to 4.5% of our waking hours. What we do in the remainder of our waking hours becomes very important in terms of calorie utilization, since most of us do not hunt and gather or till the fields. We need to build physical activity into our daily lives in simple ways, such as walking to the office next door instead of phoning, using the stairs instead of the escalator, parking further away from our destinations, walking to a more distant bus stop, or walking to the store instead of driving.

Urban planning needs to take into consideration that we need to be able to walk safely in pleasant surroundings, cycle or walk to stores and community centers, and walk safely to schools. Many parents are afraid to let their children walk to school for safety reasons, or even play outside without adult supervision.

Many residential suburban housing developments have been built in such a way that there is no alternative but to drive to the nearest mall to shop.

Treating obesity is very difficult as it is a very complex disease. I believe that we need to do more to prevent it from occurring in the first place, and that is really what I have been talking about to this point.

There are myriad different opinions and plans proposed for treating obesity, and a multimillion-dollar business in fad diets. It is estimated that Americans spend 50 billion dollars on weight loss products annually.

There are numerous fad diets such as Atkins, South beach, Zone, cabbage soup, banana, etc. Some such as Nutri System provide pre-packaged foods and others such as Bernstein are clinic based. There are well over one hundred diets that one can choose from It seems to me that if any of them really worked long term, we would not need the others. Many of the diets claim rapid weight loss in the excess of 4 to 5 pounds per week. When one realizes that one pound of fat contains 3,500 calories it is hard to see how a weight loss of that magnitude is possible, unless some of the weight loss is due to water loss.

Using the Harris Benedict equation we can estimate a person's basal metabolic rate (BMR) from the following formulae:

Men.	BMR = 66 (b.2 x Wt) + (12.7 x Ht) - (6.8 x Age)
Women.	BMR = 655 + (4.3 x Wt) + (4.7 x Ht) - (4.7 x Age)

Calorie requirements can then be estimated from the BMR depending on activity level.

Sedentary.	BMR x 1.2
Lightly active.	BMR x 1.375
Moderately active.	BMR x 1.55
Very active.	BMR x 1.725.
Athlete	BMR x 1.9

An average person weighing 70Kg requires about 1680 calories at rest per day, and if they are moderately active, would require about 2600 calories per day to maintain weight. Therefore if that moderately active person took in no calories for a day, they would in fact burn only .75

pounds of fat, and if that person took no food for one week, they would burn 5.25 pounds of fat. This means that in order to lose 5 pounds of fat in one week a person would have to be moderately active and eat nothing, which seems to me to be unlikely. As the fat is burned, water will also be lost so that the weight loss might indeed exceed 5 pounds but it cannot all be attributed to fat loss, and a slower weight loss is in my opinion more desirable.

I do not subscribe to the idea of "a diet," but believe that the best approach is healthy eating, along with sufficient exercise and sleep.

There has been much research on, and discussion in the literature, about the effects of exercise on weight loss. The consensus seems to be that while exercise is important, especially for the maintenance of weight loss, it does not cause much weight loss in and of itself.

I would argue that that is due to an insufficient dose, and will back up that point of view by referring to a study I did some years ago when I worked with a woman who ran across Canada from St. John's, Newfoundland, to Victoria, British Columbia, in 112 days. She lost 16.7 Kg (36.7 lbs) while consuming approximately 4,000 calories per day, and running 38.8 miles per day. I do recognize that it is not practical to expect people to run for eight to nine hours per day, but the point is that if the dose of exercise is high enough, weight loss can be quite significant even when calorie intake is high. In days gone by eight hours of manual labor was quite common. There are some people such as Mennonite men who continue to do many hours of physical labor on a daily basis, and I cannot recall seeing an obese Mennonite male.

The best approach for the future is to prevent our children from becoming obese, as it is very difficult to treat obesity once it is established. Unfortunately exercise is not sufficiently promoted at an early age. Insufficient attention to physical education and extracurricular sports in our schools is a problem. Thirty minutes of physical education a day with the regular classroom teacher is insufficient for health. We need to have dedicated physical education teachers in our schools, and at least an hour per day of vigorous physical activity. If we take note of what Dr. Ratey has reported in his book *Spark,* the extra time would be more than compensated for by enhanced concentration and learning in the remaining school time.

A study done at the University of Wisconsin took fifty obese, 12-year-old children and randomized them to a life style fitness orientated gym class or a standard gym class for nine months. The gym time was the same, but the experimental class had a specially trained teacher. After nine months the experimental group had lost significantly more weight, were significantly fitter and were significantly more insulin sensitive than the regular gym class group.

In addition, we as parents need to spend time in physical activity with our children when they are not in school, as well as pay attention to what they eat and drink. Cans of pop contain many empty calories, and are best avoided along with fast foods.

Lastly we need to be aware of the link between obesity and the hours of sleep. Those getting the fewest hours having a higher incidence of obesity than those getting more hours.

Unfortunately there is already an epidemic of obese people and we have to address this problem. Most people who decide to do something about their excess weight address only one side of the energy equation, the input side, and hence the interest in "diets." In order to be successful, both sides of the equation need to be dealt with, especially since the root cause of the problem for most people, has more to do with the output side of the equation than the input side. Weight loss secondary to reduced input without exercise, causes loss of both muscle and fat. Muscle burns more calories than fat, so by reducing muscle mass we further reduce the number of calories required, and make ongoing weight loss even more difficult to achieve.

In my study of obese cardiac patients, we were able to achieve a weight loss of 4.56 Kg (10 lbs) without dietary restriction, by increasing walking from a starting point of 20 minutes to 43 minutes daily over three months, and then maintaining 43 minutes of daily walking for nine more months. Body composition was determined by underwater weighing, and showed a loss of body fat mass with no change in lean body mass. We also measured resting oxygen intake, and noted an increase from 3.1 ml.kg.min at the start of the study, to 3.4 ml.kg.min at the end of the study.

Body composition is more important than weight, and I have had patients who have changed their body composition even though they did not lose weight following increased physical exertion.

I ran a pilot program in a large industrial plant where there were a high proportion of middle-aged males with trunkal obesity. They were provided with pedometers, and recorded their total daily steps for one week. After the first week they were asked to increase their total daily steps by 10% every month for six months, with a goal of reaching 10,000 steps per day. We recorded and monitored their waist circumference, weight, and blood pressure every month. The results after six months were remarkable. Waist circumference was decreased by up to 6 cm, some lost several pounds, and systolic blood pressure was reduced by up to 10 mm Hg., even though few of them reached the goal of 10,000 steps per day.

The exercise does not have to be high intensity. In fact

low intensity exercise is probably better for weight loss, and is more likely to be adhered to by the overweight person. The greater the duration, the more fat will be burned as the glycogen stores become depleted, and the body turns to utilizing triglyceride for fuel. The body becomes better able to utilize triglycerides as it becomes more accustomed to exercise.

We cannot ignore the intake side of the equation as it undoubtedly has a part to play in the obesity epidemic. There are in my view three aspects to the intake side, first the type of food ingested, secondly the portion size, and thirdly the timing of ingestion. Clearly a high fat diet will contain large numbers of calories. For instance a Big Mac with fries has approximately 700 calories, and add to that about 200 calories in a can of pop, and we are getting close to half of the days calorie requirements. Compare that to 4 ounces of salmon, a cup of broccoli, a cup of carrots and a baked potato for about 350 calories. For most people counting calorie is tedious and difficult. The simple way to eat well is to have a piece of meat or fish the size of a pack of playing cards (4 ounces), and 3 cups or more of vegetables per serving.

Portion size is a problem, especially when eating in a restaurant. Over the last number of years the plates have become larger and the serving sizes obscene. It is no wonder that we have a problem when restaurants serve 16 and 20-ounce steaks to patrons who endeavor to, and often succeed in eating them.

Timing of ingestion can make a difference. If we ate the entire day's food in one meal once a day, we would use fewer calories than if we spread the food out into three or more equal portions to be taken throughout the day. The reason is that when we eat we have to activate enzyme systems to digest the food, and that requires energy. If this happens once a day instead of several times a day, less energy is required.

People who skip breakfast, have a snack for lunch and a large dinner are more likely to have a weight problem than people who eat three meals a day. On the other hand snacking between meals requires that those calories be counted as part of the daily allowance.

Sleep deprivation in my opinion also has a part to play, not only by altering glucose metabolism, leptin and ghrelin levels, but also by providing more time in which people are likely to snack,. Television watching has been shown, particularly in children, to be associated with increased snacking on "junk" food. Some have attributed this to the advertising of inappropriate foods on children's programs.

A very recent study published in the *International Journal of Obesity* has found that attention deficit hyperactivity disorder (ADHD) is very common in obese people. Obesity in these people does not seem to respond to treatment unless the ADHD is treated first. The authors state that ADHD should be considered as a primary cause of weight loss failure in obese individuals, and that individuals seeking medical or surgical weight loss should be evaluated for ADHD and treated appropriately before intervention.

Exercise a minimum of one hour each day, the more the better.
Eat a low fat diet and watch portion control.
Eat three meals a day.
Have fruit or vegetables for snacks and limit television viewing.
Get eight hours of sleep per night.

6
Toxins

The most obvious and prevalent toxin is tobacco. Tobacco smoke contains several thousand chemicals, most of which are toxic to the body and injurious to health.

Nicotine is a compound that increases HR and BP while constricting blood vessels. Normally when HR and BP increase as the result of exercise, blood vessels dilate to allow for an increase in blood flow to accommodate the increase in energy production, and demand for oxygen by the heart muscle.

Carbon monoxide (the gas in car exhaust that can kill people) is another chemical present in cigarette smoke. Carbon monoxide combines with the red part of blood (hemoglobin) 200 times more readily than oxygen, thereby displacing oxygen. Smoking twenty cigarettes per day reduces the amount of oxygen in the blood by about 10%. Since blood now carries less oxygen, the heart has to pump more blood through narrowed vessels, against a higher pressure, to get oxygen to the tissues.

Other chemicals in cigarette smoke are known to damage the lining cells of blood vessels and promote the development of antherosclerosis. Cigarette smoke also contains chemicals that promote tongue, throat and lung cancer, but in spite of all of the above, people continue to smoke. Part of the problem is that nicotine is highly addictive, and is thought to have the same addictive propensity as cocaine. If you smoke tobacco, the single most effective thing you can do for your health is to get help in quitting.

Hormones, Antibiotics and Other Chemicals

Recombivent Bovine Growth Hormone (rBGH) is a genetically engineered hormone that is injected into dairy cows to stimulate increased milk production. It has the unfortunate side effect of increasing mastitis in the dairy cows, which in turn is treated with antibiotics, the residues of which remain in the milk. Luckily for us its use is not approved in Canada.

There are six growth hormones that are used in beef production, three naturally occurring and three synthetic. The naturally occurring ones are oestradiol, progesterone and testosterone, and the three synthetic ones are zeranol, trenbolone, and melengestrol. There has been considerable controversy at Health Canada concerning pressure by managers on scientists to approve growth hormones for use in food production. In April 1999 the European Union audited Canada's meat supply and revealed "serious deficiencies." It documented widespread use of hormones, antibiotics, endocrine disruptors and other hormonally active substances, all of which are banned in Europe. Some of the chemicals used are suspected of being linked to breast, prostate and colon cancer.

A report in the *Canadian Medical Journal* of April 2009 indicated that Canadian farmers import an estimated $100 million worth of drugs from around the world, including drugs not approved for use in Canada. These drugs include antibiotics that are given to healthy animals either to accelerate growth or to prevent infections. The concern among medical microbiologists is that some of these antibiotics are reserved for difficult to treat infections in humans, and by using them in healthy animals, the germs may develop resistance to the antibiotic and be of no use when needed for treatment of an infection in human patients.

All sorts of prescription drugs including antidepressants, antibiotics and hormones get into ground water, and to some extent into our streams, rivers, lakes and even drinking water. The risks or safety of this situation is not fully known, but the recent E Coli contamination of the Walkerton water supply should be a wake-up call as to what can happen. Walkerton is a small town in Ontario with a population of approximately 5,000 people. Their water supply became contaminated with E Coli from cattle manure, causing approximately 2,500 people to become ill and seven to die.

Bisphenol A is a chemical used in the manufacture of a wide range of consumer products such as plastic food and beverage containers, plastic food wrap, and resins that line metal cans containing food. It is a hormone disruptor and is absorbed into the body when it leaches out into water or food in contact with it, interfering with the normal functioning of the hormone system. The Canadian government is presently investigating its potentially harmful effects, and will be monitoring 5,000 Canadians as part of a health measures survey. In the meantime we would be well advised to avoid plastic water bottles and canned food. Glass or stainless steel containers are recommended as an alternative.

Heavy metals particularly lead and mercury are also found in soil and water, and mercury in large predator fish. Pesticides on food are also a concern unless the food is organically grown.

Some toxic chemicals such as acrylamide, advanced glycation end products (AGE) and polycyclic aromatic hydrocarbons (PAH) are formed during cooking.

Acrylamide is a chemical used in the production of plastics and is carcinogenic. It is formed during the cooking of plant-based foods rich in carbohydrates and low in protein at very high temperatures. Potato chips and French fries are the two foods that contain the highest levels of acrylamide. The risk to humans due to ingestion is unknown at this time, but ongoing research will likely give us answers in the future. In the meantime these are two foods that we can well do without, or at least eat in minimal quantities.

AGE are formed when meat is grilled at high temperatures on the barbecue, and are thought to promote inflammatory changes within the body. One way to minimize their formation is to cook at lower temperatures and to maintain moisture by wrapping the food in tin foil.

PAH are formed when meat is grilled to the point where there are blackened grill marks on the meat. The blackened parts should be discarded, as PAH are carcinogenic.

The green, germinating parts of potatoes contain a chemical called solanine that is toxic when ingested. It is the same chemical that is present in Deadly Nightshade. Symptoms of solanine poisoning include nausea, diarrhea, vomiting, stomach cramps, burning in the throat, heart rhythm disturbance, headache and dizziness.. The green pigment in the potato is actually chlorophyll, but its presence indicates the buildup of solanine, and the green parts of the potato should be removed, or the potato discarded. Green tomatoes also contain solanine, and should not be eaten before they ripen.

Many of the toxins to which we are exposed are used to produce the food that we eat, and are present in very small quantities, the significance of which is to some extent unknown. It may turn out that the benefits outweigh the risks, but it makes sense to minimize our exposure until the risks are quantified.

Stop smoking and avoid inhaling smoke.
Wrap foods to be barbecued in foil and discard blackened portions.
Avoid foods cooked at very high temperatures.
Limit consumption of large predatory fish.

7
Getting Started

To quote Confucius, "A journey of a thousand miles begins with a single step." Taking that first step is often the most difficult part of the journey.

Prochaska and colleagues at the University of Rhode Island developed the transtheoretical model for change in 1977. In this model, change is a "process involving progress through a series of six stages." It is worth looking at this model, to see where you are in terms of readiness to change.

Stage 1. Precontemplation. Not intending to make any changes in the foreseeable future.
Stage 2. Contemplation, Intending to make a change within the next six months.
Stage 3. Preparation. Planning to take action within the next month.
Stage 4. Action. Have made changes within the last six months.
Stage 5. Maintenance. Working to prevent relapse, from six months to five years.
Stage 6. Termination. Zero temptation to relapse, with 100% self-efficacy.

Whichever stage a person is in, the goal is to move to the next stage, until the desired change is made and becomes permanent. It is always a good idea to work on one change at a time, and to set realistic achievable goals. If you try to change too many things at once, or try to make too big a change a one time, the chances of failure become very high.

One way to minimize the difficulty of making significant change and reduce the risk of failure is to apply the principles of Kaizen—taking small steps for continuous improvement. This technique was developed during the Second World War to increase the production of war materials in the factories of America, and after the war was adopted by the Japanese in their industrial enterprises.

Telling a sedentary person to go out and do thirty minutes of moderately vigorous physical activity on a daily basis is not likely to achieve the desired result. Persuading that person to take a five-minute stroll around the block each evening, and over time to increase the length of time, distance and speed in very small increments will likely succeed without much resistance. Success generates confidence and a sense of accomplishment that encourages further change.

Change for most of us is a scary thing and that is what makes it difficult to accomplish. I remember when at the age of sixty-two I changed my career to a totally different environment, I was very uncomfortable for the first few months and wondered if I had made the right move. Over time I came to enjoy the new position even though it was a paradigm shift for me.

In his book *The Kaizen Way,* Robert Maurer explains it this way:

> Large change ⇒ fear ⇒ access to thinking part of brain restricted ⇒ failure.
> Small change ⇒ fear bypassed ⇒ thinking brain engaged ⇒ success.

It is possible to make large changes all at once, but it is much more difficult to do than to make many small changes over time. If you are someone that has had difficulty making and sticking to changes in the past, I would recommend that you pick small enough goals that you cannot fail. After achieving each goal, it becomes easier to achieve the next one and many small changes soon add up to large changes, achieved painlessly.

The first thing to do is to decide what it is that you want to change, and why you want to change it.

If you think that you need to get more sleep, keep a diary of the time that you go to bed and get up, noting how you feel when you awaken, and whether you needed an alarm to wake you. Make a note of how often you feel like napping, or actually take a nap through the day. This should quickly make you aware of any sleep deficit, and help you to decide whether or not you want to do something about it.

There are two simple questionnaires that can be used to assess for sleep deprivation. The Epworth Sleepiness Scale developed by Dr. Murray John in Melbourne, Australia, and the STOP Questionnaire developed by Dr. Francis Chung, an anesthesiologist in Toronto, Canada. (See Appendix 1 and 2).

If you think that you have a sleep disorder, make an appointment to see your doctor, but if you are just not getting enough sleep and plan to change that, remember to set a small enough goal that you know you can achieve it.

If you think that you might need to improve your diet, a good way too start is to write down everything that you eat and drink for a week. This exercise will quickly point out the areas that require attention. Again set a small goal, perhaps something as simple as cutting out a can of pop and replacing it with a glass of water, or replacing a cookie with an apple.

To get started with increasing physical activity, buy a pedometer to measure how many steps you take in a day. Record seven consecutive days so that you include a weekend, then try increasing your daily step count by 10%. If you are getting only about 4,000 steps per day or less which is quite common for a sedentary person, try increasing the number of daily steps by 10%. This amounts to an extra 400 steps per day, which is a very achievable goal. After several weeks try to increase by 10% again, gradually working your way up to 10,000 steps a day.

Another fun way to increase your physical activity is dog walking, beneficial to both you and the dog. In Indianapolis there is a program called "Walk a hound, lose a pound." Volunteers walk dogs from the animal shelter, thereby having fun while benefiting both the animal and themselves, without having to own it. Volunteers often become attached to the dog, and end up adopting it, a win-win situation for everyone.

Before starting to increase your physical activity, especially if you do so by walking, make sure that you have appropriate foot wear, and suitable clothing for seasonal outdoor activities.

Good running shoes or walking shoes are a must, and I like a sock with plenty of cushioning. It is a good idea to go to a running store to buy the shoes, as there are many different types to suit different feet and ankles. Usually the staff in running shops is experienced in what different people require in a shoe.

In cold weather, dress in layers. The layer next to your skin should be polypropylene. This material has the ability to wick away moisture without becoming wet. Wool is a good second layer and the outer layer should be waterproof, windproof and warm. Gortex meets these requirements, but is very expensive. It is always better to be too warm than too cold, as you can take layers off as needed.

A balaclava is needed for temperatures below zero, as it can cover the mouth and nose and protect you from having to breathe very cold air.

In hot weather shorts and a tee shirt are fine, but remember to cover exposed skin with sunblock if you plan to be outside for more than a few minutes, and wear a hat with a broad brim or cap with a large peak.

I had the good fortune to be in London in 1948, and saw Fanny Blankers-Koen win four track and field gold medals, 100 meters, 200 meters, 80 meters hurdles and the 4 x 100 meter relay. She was thirty years old, had two children, and could likely have won more medals, but the Olympic rules at that time limited her to four events. She was my inspiration, and I started running to the newsagent every morning to pick up the newspapers for the people with whom I was staying, and have only stopped running for one brief period of internship since. I hope that you too will find inspiration and SEE your way to better health.

Identify what you want to change.
Set small goals that you know you can achieve.
Every time you achieve your goal set a new one.

Appendix 1

STOP Questionnaire.

1. Snoring
Do you snore loudly (louder than talking or loud enough to be heard through closed doors)?

Yes No

2. Tired
Do you often feel tired, fatigued, or sleepy during daytime?

Yes No

3. Observed
Has anyone observed you stop breathing during sleep?

Yes No

4. Blood Pressure
Do you have or are you being treated for high blood pressure?

Yes No

A score of 2 or greater is high risk. When added with the criteria listed below the risk is even higher.

Neck circumference > 40 cm = 1

BMI > 35 = 1
Age > 50 = 1
Male = 1

Chung F. et al. *Anesthesiology*. 2008 May; 108 (5):812–21

Appendix 2

Epworth Sleepiness Scale

How likely are you to doze off or fall asleep in the following situations, in contrast to just feeling tired? This refers to your usual way of life in recent times. Even if you have not done some of these things recently try to work out how they would have affected you. Use the following scale to choose the most appropriate number for each situation.

0 = would never doze
1 = slight chance of dozing
2 = moderate chance of dozing
3 = high chance of dozing
(Answer each question 0, 1, 2 or 3)

Situation	Chance of dozing
1. Sitting and reading	__________
2. Watching television	__________
3. Sitting, inactive in a public place (e.g., a theatre or meeting)	__________
4. As a passenger in a car for an hour without a break	__________

5. Lying down to rest in the afternoon when circumstances permit ________
6. Sitting and talking to someone ________
7. Sitting quietly after a lunch without alcohol ________
8. In a car, while stopped for a few minutes in traffic ________

Score	
1–6	Congratulations, you are getting enough sleep.
7–8	Your score is average
9–24	Seek the advice of a sleep specialist without delay

Johns M.W., *Sleep,* 1991 Dec; 14 (6):540-5

Further Reading

Sleep Thieves Stanley Coren, Published by Simon and Schuster
Fats that Heal and Fats that Kill Udo Erasmus. Alive Books
Textbook of Work Physiology Per-Olof Astrand, Karrre Rodahl. McGraw-Hill
Walking, Weight and Wellness Martin Collis. Trafford Publishing
Take Heart Terence Kavanagh. Key Porter Books
Spark John J. Ratey. Little, Brown and Company
The Kaizen Way Robert Maurer. Workman Publishing